See the Best in You

Tips and guidelines to achieve beautiful, flawless skin

Dr Shiv Dua

An imprint of
B. Jain Publishers (P) Ltd.
An ISO 9001 : 2000 Certified Company
USA — EUROPE — INDIA

Information given in this book is not intended to be taken as a replacement for medical advice. Any person with a condition requiring medical attention should consult a qualified medical practitioner. The comments and treatments suggested by the author are his views and publishers need not agree with him.

SEE THE BEST IN YOU

First Edition: 2011
1st Impression: 2011

All rights reserved. No part of this book may be reproduced, stored in a retrieval system or transmitted, in any form or by any means, mechanical, photocopying, recording or otherwise, without any prior written permission of the publisher.

© with the publisher

Published by Kuldeep Jain for

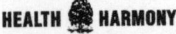

An imprint of
B. JAIN PUBLISHERS (P) LTD.
An ISO 9001 : 2000 Certified Company
1921/10, Chuna Mandi, Paharganj, New Delhi 110 055 (INDIA)
Tel.: +91-11-4567 1000 • *Fax:* +91-11-4567 1010
Email: info@bjain.com • *Website:* **www.bjain.com**

Printed in India by
J.J. Offset Printers

ISBN: 978-81-319-0861-7

Foreword

Dr Shiv Dua has requested me to write a foreword for his new book on care of skin and beauty. It has been my pleasure to go through the manuscript of the book and I found it quite interesting. The basic aim of the book appears to be the care of skin through alternative therapies like diet control, yoga, herbal aids, change of life style and of course, homeopathic medicines. The book has 'management' as its unique feature to cure certain skin disorders. The problem with such type of books is that they often do not lay sufficient emphasis on the disease-states and medical terminology peculiar to the tropical countries and especially common in India. To overcome this weakness and make it the strength of the book, Dr Dua has amalgamated both medical terminology and non-medical simple methods for the care of skin. He has also detailed the harms of cheap cosmetics, harsh sunlight, frost bite, dry or oily skin and all basic knowledge about the various skin conditions for better understanding of the common man.

I have seen some of his previous books on thyroid, cervical spondylosis, kidney and gall bladder stones, hernia, hair care and nails care etc. The general outlay and common feature of all these books is to impart basic knowledge about the diseases with 'management' through alternative therapies including homeopathy. However, it would have been more interesting had there been pictorial view of the cases with illustrations showing clinical improvements. The success of such 'managing' of diseases in his books is evident by the fact that four of his books have been translated into Spanish and one book is translated into Russian.

I wish this publication a wide readership and patronage.

Dr Malkit Singh
MD (Dermatology), A.I.I.M.S., New Delhi.

Preface

From time immemorial, the care of skin has been under strict surveillance of people of all races of all countries. India has a history of beautiful women and handsome men. The idols in our holy temples speak of our aesthetic background. The concern for beautiful skin is also revealed in the legendry religious books. Since ages, women have been striving to achieve a beautiful and fabulous skin and for this they have been searching for new methods differently in each era. They have been adopting various methods to improve upon their complexion by using different applicants, both domestic and herbal, available in the particular era in which they lived.

Today the scenario is not much different. Most of the women in cities and small towns head for shops that sell beauty products. Beauty business today is dynamic and experimental. New products, innovations, and techniques are being introduced in the market continuously. I was drawn to the subject of the book due to the increasing demand of beauty products in the market. Even the most common 'Mehndi' (henna, used widely in India) has become a favourite tool of beauty.

Rising income of young ambitious girls and women working in multinational companies and call centres have cultivated their interest in personal grooming. The growing interest to look good and feel fit is universal. In this respect, even the non-working women living in common social stature with families are addicted to visit beauty salons every month. The awareness is so acute that even little girls want their part of beauty job to be done in salons. Everyone knows that looking good and being fit has a deep connection with routine exercise and a nutritional diet. But sadly enough, people have no time for all this. They go for the easiest solution, which is the use of cosmetics. Cosmetics available in the market give temporary glow to the outward look. In the long run they harm the skin. Many beauty products do not suit the texture of the skin. One should have knowledge of one's skin and use cosmetics only after that. In general, people know about two types of skin—oily and dry. Rarely do people know about the third type of skin which is the 'mixed' type.

This book guides the readers about the secrets and the type of skin they possess. Once the texture of the skin is known, it becomes easy to use proper cosmetics without any harm. In most of the beauty products, there is information about the suitability of the product for dry, oily or mixed skin.

We are at present living in a world of glamour and are very conscious about our appearances (skin). Beauty salons or health resorts are in plenty in big cities and people are utilizing the same. We spend money, time, gadgets, tools and medicines to create the required change in our appearance. The obese wish to be slim and the ugly wish to be beautiful. On one side, the age factor is bent upon making an impact on the skin and on the other side, the women are persistently taking help of the means that can make them appear young. All types of aesthetic treatments promote a sense of well-being. The quality of beauty resorts should have aestheticians who are intelligent, caring and qualified to give you a well-groomed appearance. Those who cannot afford to go to beauty parlours or resorts, naturally depend on the beauty products available in the market. Recently the word 'herbal' has become a obsession. Most of the products sell hot due to their herbal contents. What are these herbs?

Preface

How has aloe vera come into the limelight and what are its actual uses? It is all explained in this book. Not only females are attracted towards the world of cosmetics, the males are the latest targets. Males have become pretty conscious about their appearances nowadays.

This trend has triggered the onset of many beauty products suitable for males. It is the urban male population which is more interested in the products. Gone are the days when males did not much care about their appearance. Today's men want to look good all the time. This book has tips for males too to look beautiful.

There is no doubt that good nutrition, a healthy living style and physical exercise results in excellent texture and glow on the skin. Together, all these factors keep the body strong to fight the age-related skin disorders and diseases. The variety of foods that we take, the environment we live in and the life style we maintain, directly surfaces on our skin and changes it to a fabulous one or a dull and dreary one. This angle of life in skin changes have been discussed in this book. Maintaining skin health through sound sleep, constipation free body, freshening baths, tensionless brains with 'Yoga' are also detailed in the book.

In the recent times, plastic surgery is becoming very popular among the people of the higher society who are rich and affluent. Erasing wrinkles, lifting the nasal shape, straightening angle of chin or cheeks, up-lifting breasts etc. are common corrections that people seek from plastic surgeons. It is up to the choice of the person to opt surgery. But the most common thing that everybody seems to be interested in is 'Botox' by which wrinkles are erased. What is Botox and what are its advantages or disadvantages? This book has its easy explanation to this as well. I hope this book will help all those interested in modern beauty therapy.

Shiv Dua

Acknowledgements

- Mr Kuldeep Jain, Proprietor, CEO, M/s B. Jain Publishers, New Delhi for his continued support to me in writing books.
- Mr Manish Jain, Director, M/s B. Jain Publishers, New Delhi for suggesting the topic of the book in our meeting during 'Author's presence and consultations with the readers/patients' session at the 'World Book Fair, New Delhi' on 5th Feb. 08.
- Dr Ravinder Kochhar, Principal, LMHM College, Ludhiana. Meeting him and listening to his lectures on skin injuries in the seminar (Feb., 08) was an inspiration to me.
- Dr Jinesh Kumar Jain, President, Northern India Homoeopathic Chemists Association, Ludhiana for his invitation to the seminar in (Feb., 08) enabled me to learn a lot. His lecture on surgery without knife was a noble tribute to homoeopathy.
- Dr Geeta, Editor, The Homoeopathic Heritage, for her valuable inputs for the work.
- Dr Sanjeev Kumar, BHMS, Gold medallist, Faridabad for providing literature on the subject and purposeful discussions on the subject.
- Dr Lalit Aggarwal for giving valuable hints on homoeopathic literature on skin. His initiative to continue and initiate scientific meetings of the doctors of Faridabad is valuable.

- Dr Pravesh Aggarwal, Palwal, for his help in writing this book.

- Mr Yash Pal Shahi, Shastri Nagar, Model Town, Ludhiana for his kind hospitality during my stay with him and suggesting me to write this book on beauty and skin.

- My old seniors and friends of Geological Survey of India, Shri M.C. Appa, V.G. Rajagopalan, R. Krishnan, C.L. Rajendra Kumar, and C. V. Rajaiah. Their messages of encouragement instilled moral strength in me to write.

- My family members Uma, Dharmesh, Anuradha, Amit, Nilima, Tanya, Akshay and Aryan for helping in writing the book.

- Dr Malkit Singh, MBBS, MD (AIIMS), Skin and VD specialist of Faridabad for his help in explaining difficult definitions of skin diseases. His support to homoeopathy in certain types of skin diseases is appreciated.

Publisher's Note

It is indeed a natural desire to look beautiful. A beautiful face, a vibrant body, glowing skin and fabulous health are everlasting desires of each one of us. But sadly, the modern culture of 'eat, drink and be merry' is obstructing the young to resort to the healthy living style.

Urban population today is leaning towards a culture which revolves around shopping malls and is fond of junk food and has access to all the chemicals and cosmetics which they use without hesitation. But many times, they harm rather than benefitting. When the beauty products do not fetch the desired results, they consult doctors and when this does not work too, the next step is to approach cosmetologists.

The book is a solution to all such problems of skin and beauty care which one might be looking for. This book tells about many beauty products and their correct use and also the treatment alternatives in your kitchen.

When life becomes intolerably stressful, it shows on the face. The book discusses different ways to de-stress oneself and the finer aspects of skin care. It also discusses other aspects of grooming like hair care, nail care, feet care, etc.

Dr Shiv Dua has been writing for health awareness topics since more than a decade and we are proud to have published his works. His books are in demand and many of his books have also been translated into foreign languages like Spanish, Russian and Arabic. His writings are beyond continents. We thank him again for bringing out this wonderful work on skin care.

Kuldeep Jain
C.E.O., B. Jain Publishers (P) Ltd.

About the Author

Dr Shiv Dua, M.A., D. I. Homeopathy, HMD (London) is a well-known name in the literary circle of homeopathy. His books have been published and well accepted by the readers. Some of his books have gone into repeated editions. He has written more than 190 articles on various subjects concerning homeopathy which are published in the leading hindi newspapers and english magazines. He has been delivering lectures in seminars, scientific meetings of doctor's associations and Homoeopathic Medical Colleges. Dr Dua has been awarded appreciation awards by many institutes like 'The Lions Club of Faridabad', and 'The Doctor's Associations'. He has worked in many charitable hospitals in Jaipur and Faridabad. At present, he is occupied with his academic and creative work. He has written the following books:

1. *Practitioner's guide to Gall Bladder Stones and Kidney Stones*
2. *Oral Diseases*
3. *Know and Solve your Thyroid Problems*
4. *Cervical Spondylosis-Neck pain*
5. *Constitutional Remedies through Interesting Short Stories*
6. *Homoeopathic Self-healing Guide for Beginners*
7. *Hair Care*

8. *Nails care*
9. *King Gland, Prostate*
10. *Inguinal Hernia*

Contents

Foreword .... *iii*
Preface .... *v*
Acknowledgements .... *ix*
Publisher's Note .... *xi*
About the Author .... *xiii*

Chapters

1. Think Young and be Young 1
   - Dark Complexion 2
   - Did you know? 3
   - How to Check the Texture of Your Skin? 4
   - SPF Factor and Sunscreen Creams 4
   - Ill Effects of Cosmetics 5
2. Structure, Functions and Concept of Skin and its Diseases .. 7
   - Ways of Life Today 7
   - Mixed Generation 8
   - Edible Oils and the New Generation 9
   - Cheap Cosmetics 10

- From Villages to Cities 11
- Examine your Fitness.. 12
- Fabulous Skin 13
- Skin Allergy, Bacteria and Lesions 20
- Allergy 22
- Bacteriology 25
- Classification of Lesions 26
- Classification of Primary and Secondary Lesions 34

3. Examining Skin Conditions, Texture and Health 39
   - Difference Between Skin Diseases and Skin Disorders 39
   - Parameters of Skin Disorders and Diseases 40
   - Who Possesses Healthy Skin? 44
   - Structural Difference and Skin Diseases 45
   - Structural Differences and Nature of Skin 46

4. Common Avoidable Problems of the Skin 49
   - Common Avoidable Problems 49
   - Corns 53
   - Callosities 54

5. Seven Factors that Balance the Beauty of Skin 57
   - Constipation 58
   - Hygiene 62
   - Discharges of the Body 65
   - Walking 67
   - Sleep and Rest 68

- Skin Health of Babies 71
- Stress 73
- Fasts 75
- Examining Skin Health 75
- Daily Examination of Your Body 76
- Weekly Examination of Your Body 78

6. Cosmetic Care of the Face and the Skin 81
   - Are Cosmetics Important? 81
   - Men Chase Cosmetics Too! 82
   - Which Cosmetics are the Most Used? 83
   - Side Effects of Cosmetics not Suiting the Skin 84
   - Herbal Cosmetics 84
   - Oily Skin Test 85
   - Dry Skin Test 86
   - Mixed Oily and Dry Skin Test 88
   - Healthy Skin of the Face 88
   - Massage of the Face 92
   - Facial Massage at Home 94
   - Cosmetic Care Preparations at Home for Oily Skin 97
   - Toners 99
   - Home-Made Preparations for Dry Skin 100

7. Care of Complexion 103
   - Dark Complexion and Beauty 105
   - Selection of Wrong Beauty Products 106
   - Impact of Anaemic Condition on Complexion 107

- Impact of Acne and Pimples on Complexion 107
- Impact of Poor Blood Circulation and Hormonal Disturbance 107
- Impact of Food on Complexion 107
- Sun Shine or Sunburns and Complexion 108
- Alcohol 113
- Smoking 113
- Tea or Coffee 114
- Beauty Baths 115
- Home Remedies 117
- Care of Dry Skin in Reference to Complexion 118
- Use of Soaps and Face Washes 121

8. Features that Add Beauty to the Face 125
   - Care of Teeth 125
   - Care of Neck 128
   - Care of Knees, Elbows and Ankles 129
   - Care of Hair 130
   - Care of Lips 134
   - Kajal for Your Eyes 138
   - Care of the Back 139
   - Uses of Brushes 139

9. Medical Help for Beauty 141
   - What is 'Botox'? 142

10. Nails 145
    - How are Nails Related with the Body? 146

Contents

- Diseases and Nails 147
- Nail Biting 148

11. Nine Problems of the Face 157
    - Acne and Pimples 158
    - Blackheads (Comedones) 163
    - Blemishes 167
    - Chloasma 169
    - Dark Circles 170
    - Freckles 172
    - Liver Spots or Brown Spots 173
    - Moles/Naevi 174
    - Wrinkles of Face 175
    - Warts 179

12. Hirsutism 181
    - Unwanted Hair Growth on the Face 181
    - Causes 182
    - Prognosis 183
    - Treatment 184
    - Removal of Hair 185

13. Yoga and Beauty 191
    - What is Yoga? 191
    - Pranayam, the Correct Breathing 194
    - Yoga and Skin 198
    - Sarvangasan (Standing on Shoulders) 199
    - Shavasana (Corpse Pose) 200

- Tarh-Asana 201
- Kon-Asana 201
- Bi-Weekly Body Massage 202

14. Normal Values of Weight, Height and Laboratory Findings 205
    - Normal Weight and Height Chart 206
    - Laboratory Findings 207
    - Lasting Of Diseases 209

Bibliography *211*

Chapter 1

Think Young and be Young

In this world there are people who are much concerned about the way they look. Gazing at the mirror has become a common ritual among the young. Observing a small pimple on the face disturbs them so much that they run to the Dermatologists. The reason is obviously very clear. No one likes to look ugly. Such a feeling comes from the mind. It is the mind which tells you that you are looking ugly! Try telling your friends or relatives that you have eruptions on your face. No one minutely watches that small pimple on your face. It is you who is more concerned. It is for sure that you should change such a type of thinking. You have to develop a sort of confidence that skin disorders can be cured without medicines. You have to change your life style and diet. The visit to a doctor comes at a much later stage. If you develop good and youthful thoughts, the result will also be good too.

If you go on thinking that you are getting old and will have a wrinkled skin in the near future, even at the age of forty, you will really get old. The thought that 'everyone has to get old one day' should be kept away though it is true that old age is unavoidable.

Let it dawn at its own natural pace. If you start thinking young, you will be really young.

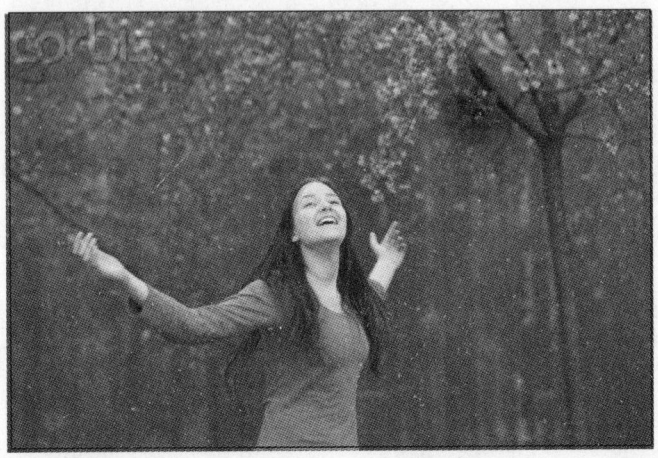

Think positive to remain beautiful

Eight Enemies of skin's complexion:

- Age (getting aged)
- Lack of sleep
- Lack of nutritional food
- Alcohol
- Smoking and chewing tobacco
- Lack of exercise
- Exposure to sunburns, and polluted environment
- Wrong life-style

DARK COMPLEXION

Complexion whether fair or dark is a gift of God. In reality beauty is distributed equally in all the complexions, be it fair or dark.

I feel that dark complexion is more attractive than the fair provided the features of the face are sharp and in the correct proportion.

Dark complexion has its own advantages. Firstly, wrinkles are seldom visible on this type of complexion. The sun burns are lesser than the fair faces. The muscles of a dark face are much stronger than those of a fair face. And the greatest advantage of a dark face is that the process of ageing is much slow!

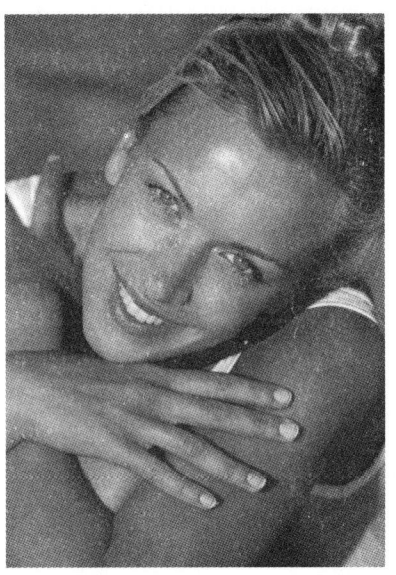

A dusky beauty

DID YOU KNOW?

- Not drying the skin after taking bath and wearing clothes over wet skin is equivalent to inviting skin infections.
- Lack of sleep and rest can result in dusky complexion and dark rings beneath and around the eyes.
- Covering the face with bed sheet or blanket while sleeping may ruin the complexion and texture of the face.
- Constipation triggers lackluster skin (lacking brightness).
- Improper and inferior quality face creams and creams not in tune with oily or dry skin may harm the face and its texture.
- Sunlight exposure, frostbite, corns, callosities and shoe blisters also causes damage to the skin though temporarily. The skin returns to its normal texture even without medicines provided timely care is taken.

- Visiting your friends or relatives admitted in the hospital's ICU wards without wearing a mask (face cover cloth) on the face is inviting infectious diseases. Such visits could also trigger or increase facial acne or pimples.
- Anxiety, fear, repressed anger and emotions lead to many skin diseases.

HOW TO CHECK THE TEXTURE OF YOUR SKIN?

Take some tissue paper. Fold it in strips. In the early morning without washing your face, rub and slide the strips to and fro gently over your nose, forehead, chin, and cheeks. Now check the strip. If there are some stains of grease, your skin is oily. If there are no stains and the strips remain unchanged, your skin is dry. Next morning without washing the face, rub and slide a strip on the centre of your face starting from you forehead to nose and chin. See the strip.

Now take another strip and rub/slide it on the cheeks and the surrounding areas. Check the strip.

In the above two tests, if the results differ from each other, that means that the central part of your face is oily and the sides are dry. You have a mixed skin.

SPF FACTOR AND SUNSCREEN CREAMS

Every onset of summer brings in loads of sunscreen creams and all the cosmetic manufacturers are generally very proud about these creams. Every good cream has a logo of sun protection factor (SPF) written on its product. SPF is a measuring unit to combat sunshine. It is useful armament to judge the capacity to fight against sunshine in USA and Europe. This awareness is gaining momentum in India too. The skins of the Indians have sufficient pigments to fight the harmful effects of the ultraviolet rays of sun. It is also susceptible to tanning but it never burns the skin as experienced in USA or Europe. This is the reason that skin cancer in India is very rare!

ILL EFFECTS OF COSMETICS

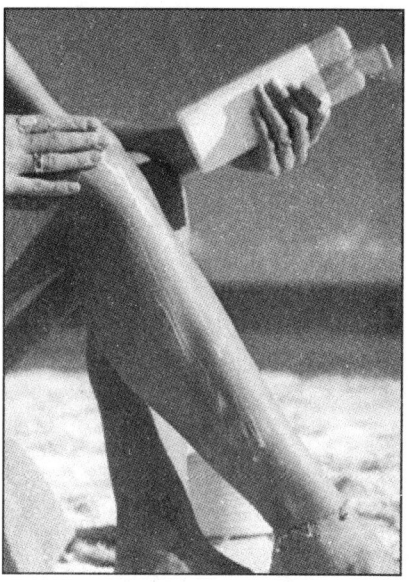

Sunscreen creams save you

People in general have a tendency to purchase the advertised cosmetics for acne and other skin problems. In case, if these cosmetics do not suit the skin of the buyer, the harm done by the product to the skin will be more than its benefits. In such cases, the use of the particular cosmetic/cream, lotion should be discontinued at once. An effective remedy in removing the evil effects of cosmetics is taking Bovista 30, a homoeopathic medicine, 4 pills three times a day for seven days.

Chapter 2

Structure, Functions and Concept of Skin and its Diseases

WAYS OF LIFE TODAY

It is indeed ironical that no human being on earth wants death although we know that it is imminent. Everyone desires to live for hundred of years that too in good health. Most of us wish to complete the circle of age as per the legendary 'Vedic' books and everyone desires to live for 100 years, if not 108 years, the stipulated complete life of a perfect human being. But sadly, there is a lot of difference between wishing and achieving. To accomplish the much desired wish, one has to set a goal for oneself and act according to that plan of achieving. This goal of health and longevity is not materialistic like having ambitions of acquiring service, building a home, or fulfilling an academic achievement etc. Along with this first desire is to live long there is always a second longing desire in every person.

The second strong irresistible desire is to look beautiful and attractive. This second desire can only be fulfilled if life fulfils certain conditions like the home-atmosphere should be peaceful, environment should be pollution-free, water should be worth drinking, eatables nutritious, habits should not be bad and the temperament is adjustable.

The villages and remote places in the lap of nature do fulfill some of the above aspects but a grave drawback is their poverty. It is due to this that the skin of villagers becomes devoid of glow. Another drawback to achieve sound skin-texture in villages is the lack of adequate health education. If they are ignorant about the maintenance of health, taking timely treatment and knowing the disease, the whole purpose of looking beautiful is lost. If they consult witch doctors, the skin health maybe ruined. The people of the urban world have an edge over the rural population where education is concerned and they have medical facilities at hand also to deal with the diseases of skin on time.

MIXED GENERATION

Gone are the days when our older generation was aware of the old traditions of living-style. They used to give advices to the young generation about health rules. We in India had joint families and the elders noted even the slightest thing going wrong with skin. They did not hesitate even for a minute to suggest remedial measures for such ailments and the members of family had no hesitation to follow the instructions of elders as well. But now the things have changed. The new generation has taken over. They believe in the half-modern and half-traditional way of living.

This new generation has been brought up in a changed style of living where science rules with the invasion of transistors, MP-3, mobiles, computers, movies, digital cameras and televisions. The modern era which is loaded with gadgets has given way to a new life style that has advantages and disadvantages. The advertisements of the media are both beneficial and useless. Instead of a simple breakfast, the young generation feels encouraged eating bread and its products. The advertisements have changed the strict vegetarian families into non-vegetarians inspiring them to eat at least eggs. Bread, Maggie, tomato sauce, jams, pizza, burger, cold drinks, and use of synthetic solvents in milk have taken over the old menu even in the shops of small towns.

The market of small towns and big villages are now flooded with scented oils, tooth pastes, scented soaps, cheap creams, shampoos and cosmetics to convert dark complexion into a fair one.

This type of a mixed generation who is neither 'modern' nor 'outmoded' often falls pray to cheap advertised cosmetics that ruins their skin's health. This generation is educated and can be brought to a suitable level by making them read books that contain basic knowledge of skin.

EDIBLE OILS AND THE NEW GENERATION

Today the market is flooded with a variety of edible oils, mixed and vegetable oils (cottonseed, soya, and sunflower) because they are cheaper than our traditional oil we have been using. Our ancestors have been consuming mustard oil, groundnut oil, sesame oil and coconut oil in accordance with the tradition of their states in India and did not have serious health problems except epidemics. The media today with their powerful advertising tools have actually allured people to buy and experiment with several edible oils available in the market even if they have never used them ever in their lives! Often I get patients for treatment of skin diseases that have erupted due to the oil-use that did not suit their body. If the oil is not suiting, people get rashes and allergies, pimples or boils scattered all over the body.

Recently, a patient of mine who had red rashes and a crop of small boils spread over his arms, legs, chest and back came for a check-up. He told that this skin problem has not come alone to him but his wife and children also suffered from the same type of skin rashes. Their severity was less than his. I examined his symptoms and gave him medicine which did not work. After a fortnight of taking medicine, when I enquired about his food and cooking medium, he revealed that he was using sunflower oil since the last six months. Without consulting any doctor, he had switched over to sunflower oil as he had read in the newspapers that it was good for the heart. He also said that he had got his blood pressure checked which was on higher side. And so he himself bought the oil in the hope of decreasing his blood pressure.

I checked his B.P. It was normal. He was told to discontinue sunflower oil at once and start using mustard oil which he was taking prior to taking sunflower oil. He was given sac-lack (a medicine that has no medicinal contents) and told to report after one week. Within a week, he reported that his rashes and boils on his body had disappeared and all his family members are also cured that too without taking any medicine. I told him to get his blood pressure checked after a month. His blood pressure after a month was found to be normal without taking sunflower oil or any medicine.

One has to be careful while choosing their cooking medium if they wish to change their traditional one. No experiment should be done without the consultation of a doctor. I have seen many other cases where people have suffered due to the changing of oil.

CHEAP COSMETICS

Now let us for a moment forget the use of cooking oil and consider the use of cosmetics. Very seldom do people realise that the use of improper and cheap cosmetics may ruin their skin-health. The hair turns gray prematurely by the use of scented hair oils or the 'cool' oils which are said to be enriched with 'herbs'. The constant use of cheap quality scented body wash, deodorants, scented chemical soaps, shampoos, talcum powders, face-washes, scrubs, and after-bath cosmetics make the skin rough and may help in the eruption of rashes or allergies. Going in the sun, getting wet in the rain, excessive use of hot or cold air (when coming in or out of air-conditioned rooms) and abrupt changes in the climate make many people uneasy. Rashes or other skin ailments appear. These rashes are mostly related to skin diseases. But they are actually due to change in atmosphere. Much of this sensitiveness is due to the use of cheap cosmetics. This trend is obviously adopted by people who cannot afford good quality cosmetics in the cities. Even if they want good quality cosmetics, there are many imitations available. If one wants to purchase a bottle of 'Ponds' cream, the shopkeeper seeing the customer's lack of knowledge in these things show an imitation named 'Pands' that has same design and colour on the bottle. One should be careful to identify such duplicates.

FROM VILLAGES TO CITIES

Living a long and a healthy life in villages has become a dream because of rapid urbanization and intrusion of city-culture. In the hope of better employment, the villagers are leaving the villages and running towards cities for better occupation, better housing facilities and better education. It is a general human tendency to look towards the better things in life. The good thing in this respect is only in the 'appearance'. Whether it is really good and profitable in all respects is still a debatable question.

The world of television has reached many villages in India and has made a difference in their thinking. The irony is that the idea of leaving the villages is considered extremely profitable from the viewpoint of the villagers but it ends in the tragedy of ill health in the long run.

The simple minded villagers fail to see the negativities of urban life. They do not get fresh air, good diet, fresh milk and pollution free air to breathe to which their bodies are generally used to from birth. This is one aspect of life but the real culprit is again cosmetics. They fall a victim to cheaper quality cosmetics and imitated brands. Whether you are from a city or a village, you must know about the general fitness of the body. In very easy language this is given below for the benefit of readers.

EXAMINE YOUR FITNESS

General Fitness of the Body

General fitness of the body can be accounted by the following factors:

- Physical strength of the muscles
- The power to withstand physical exertion
- The ability to withstand the cardiac pressures (not getting easily fatigued)
- The flexibility of the body

Consider Yourself Healthy

- When you are unconscious and unaware about the act of breathing
- When you do not hear the sound of your own breathing or your heartbeats
- When your breathing is without effort

General Unfitness of the Body

- The body gets tired even when trying to board a bus or a train

- The body struggles even when climbing a slope or stairs
- The body exhausts easily while playing some physical game of sports
- The body gains weight year after year

You are not Healthy

- When you hear your breathing and you are aware of it (except while exercising, running, doing Pranayam etc.)
- When others near you hear your breathing
- When the breathing is non-rhythmic and non-methodical
- When your *body mass index and waist to tip ratio is incorrect (* See definition of body mass index and normal body weights in the last chapter of the book)

FABULOUS SKIN

In the modern era, most of the people are quite conscious of their skin and beauty. Earlier this phenomenon was mostly restricted to women only. Sensing this trend, the market is full of cosmetics for enhancing one's, beauty with natural products. This is all done to achieve a fabulous skin, gain knowledge about preservation of youthful skin and enjoy good health.

We are blessed with a human body that has an inner and outer appearance. The outer covering of a human body is the skin. Taken in its entirety, the skin is one of the biggest organs in the body. It is held responsible for many important functions. The skin has its sensation of touch and has various sensations of temperatures. This sensation is the greatest at the fingertips. The skin also protects the underlying epidermal cells from the radiation of the sun's rays.

In the inside of the body we have different organs and a beautiful interconnected system of work that makes the body alive. Inside the body, we have the basic unit of life in the forms of cells. The cells actually form the whole set up of life. It is easy to understand the formation of cells. If you put a cork under the microscope and see its magnified shape, you will find innumerable minute compartments. There are large number of units invisible to the naked eyes. These cells look completely different from one another and they perform specialized functions in particular regions of the body.

The cells of the liver and brain have different shape as they perform different jobs. So, cells make different organs and in between the organs a lot of fluid exists. This fluid is the vital food called *blood*. Blood is always moving. Then we have our life line—the lungs and the heart.

We have the kidneys, the nervous system, the endocrines, and the sexual organs depicting the cycle of life. All this is inside the body and not visible to the naked eye. What is visible is the outer layer of the body called skin. Skin acts as a wrapper of the body and it needs bathing, shaving, scratching, or anointing when dry. Actually, it is more than a wrapper. The best part of skin is that it produces vitamin 'D'. It also activates and regulates blood pressure. It stimulates the sex hormones and testerones. The best function that the skin performs is that it keeps water out and does not allow it inside the body when we take bath in a bathtub or a swimming pool. In other words, the skin is the protector of the inner organs of the body. Skin also protects against strong potential of bacteria that lives on the skin but does not enter the body.

The hair, the nails of fingers and toes and the callus on the soles and palms are part of the skin. They too protect the inner body. Skin is waterproof. Its pH on the surface varies from 4.5 to 6.5 and there is every possibility that this acid mantle has a bacterial function that is essential for well-being of the epidermis.

The skin does not dry in the heat or melt in the rains and it protects from the radiation of sunlight.

Skin is very tough against wounds and it acts as a shield against injuries. Skin also conserves heat or cools the body as needed and hence keeps the internal temperature constant. Skin is made of three layers, *epidermis* and *dermis* and *subcutaneous*.

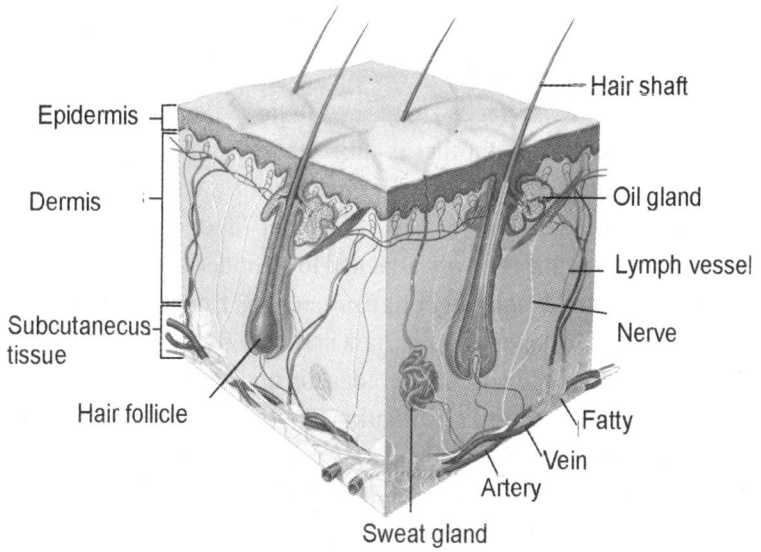

Structure of the skin

- *Epidermis* is the outermost layer of the skin
- *Dermis* is the middle layer of the skin
- *Subcutaneous* is the bottom most layer of the skin

The structural arrangements of the above layers are variable, different, and not alike but there is a close relationship between each layer. This close association ensures the unity of action of the skin. This unity is more between the outer layer and the true skin (or corium consists of fine thread-like fibers arranged in finger like elevations and depressions). It is held together by an adhesive like substance and by a series of finger like elevations and depressions. We know that every organ of the body should have blood but this epidermis of the skin is without blood vessels. If there are no blood vessels, how are they nourished? A special fluid called lymph nourishes them. Its cells are nourished by diffusion from below that is, dermis.

The epidermis consists of many layers of cells; the bottom-most are called the mother cells. These cells are constantly dividing and moving up to the surface. There they flatten, die and change into a material called keratin that is ultimately shed as tiny, invisible scales. It takes about three to four weeks for a cell in the lowest layer to reach the skin surface. The outer layer, epidermis, is a protective layer that is firmly attached to an underlying layer called dermis. Very small and finger like projections from the dermis and fit into into the socket of epidermis and this gives birth to ridges. Ridges are at the junction of epidermis and dermis. We can see these ridges or wave like formation on the fingertips, which act as fingerprints. The dermis is made of collagen and elastin fibers. In the dermis are sweat, sebaceous and apocrine glands, blood vessels, nerves and hair follicles. The blood vessels are limited in the dermis but nerves go deep into the epidermis.

The sebaceous glands open into the hair follicles and consist of specialised epidermal cells that produce sebum. They are innumerable on the face, the chest, the back and on the head. The subcutaneous part of our skin layer acts as an insulator to conserve our body heat. The function of these glands is to lubricate the hair shaft and the surrounding skin and their control is through sex hormones.

The hair can be shaved without damaging the epidermis or spilling of blood because there is no blood supply in it. Its cells are nourished by diffusion from below that is dermis. One wonders why we do not shed our skin just like the snake do. Yes, epidermis also sheds but it is a very slow process.

Everyday, millions of tiny epidermal cells are made in the innermost part of epidermis and start pushing their way outwards. When we take bath, millions of them are washed away and our skin gets renewed.

Blood Vessels

We have talked about blood vessels above. The job of blood vessels is an interesting one to note. When we exert ourselves with some work or do exercises on a hot day, these blood vessels dilate and we begin to sweat. It radiates heat to the outside to relieve the sweat. On the other hand, on a cold winter day, it is the opposite. The blood vessels close and divert the blood to the interior of the body and the skin looks pale. The blood vessels are also under the directives and commands of our emotions. When we are angry, we flush on the face, which means that the blood vessels are open. When we are frightened, our feet go cold that means the blood vessels are shut. Regarding sweat glands, we have still another interesting story to tell.

Sweat Glands

Sweat glands are located in the deepest part of the skin. Their number is more in the armpits, groins, palms and the soles. They are just like long tubes with opening on the outer skin. We have about two o three million sweat glands in our skin. Sweat glands act like air conditioners of the body. Evaporation of sweat cools the body.

If the body temperature is more than normal of 98.4 F, we experience difficult time. Sweat glands work and extract water, salt, and some wastes from the blood. While sweating, our sweat glands produce about half a kilo of water in normal temperature but while exercising, the extraction of water is much more. It is about 5 Kg. Emotions also play a role in sweat glands as they play in the case of blood vessels.

In times of anxiety and tension, we break into cold sweat because there is rapid evaporation. There will be cold sweat on the palms and the soles. There is also a close relationship between the amount of sweat secretion and the quantity of urine voided. In winter, we secrete very little or negligible sweat and the urine is more and abundant. In summer, the urine is scanty but the sweat is more. The body always maintains a normal and stipulated water-balance and anything coming in order to change this balance is fought and excess or less is brought to a balance through discharges and drinking. This is the wonder of our amazing body.

Oil Glands

Like sweat glands, we have oil glands on the true skin. Mainly they are found in hair and hair sacs but they also exist independently. These oil glands are similar in shape like the bunches of grapes in the vines and they secrete fatty material that lubricates the skin and the hair. Those who have oily skin have active oil glands and people with dry skin have inactive oil glands.

Muscles

Like sweat glands and oil glands, muscles also exist in the true skin. They are erectors of hair called 'arrectores pilorum'. The muscles start from true skin and end in the regions of many associated hair follicles. The muscles and the air sacs help expulsion of the oily secretion from the oil glands and in raising the hair.

Sebaceous Glands

Now, let us talk about sebaceous or fat glands. Situated in the third layer of the skin, they are simply masses of fat. They are hundred thousands of them on the body and as the name indicates they are glands having lot of fat in them. They produce semi-liquid oil and are mostly attached to the hair follicles. They have their own unique way of nourishing and lubricating both the hair and the surrounding skin. These glands really serve a very good purpose.

The hair is almost water proof and they have the capacity to retain heat of the body but with pollution of the atmosphere, the hair become clogged and form cellular debris or even pimples blackheads on the face. This is the reason why young men and women apply moisture-less creams on hair and face. The fat is responsible for the natural outline of the body and when a person is emaciated, this fat deposit becomes less.

Melanocytes

There are millions of cells called melanocytes on the skin. They produce the pigment called melanin. It is the pigment melanin that determines the colour of hair, the eyes and the complexion of the skin. Melanin is the protective substance that avoids dangerous ultraviolet sun's rays. When we are out in the sun, the pigment granules of the skin begin rising from the lower part of epidermis to the surface of the skin and thus protect it. A person especially ladies, getting freckles is the result of concentration of melanin on the skin.

Auto Transformation of Skin

When we are near to the age of fifty or so, our skin undergoes many changes. The skin becomes thin with the advancement of age, veins in the back of hands and arms become prominent and visible, the undercoat of fat diminishes and wrinkles form on the skin. Our elastic skin becomes loose and starts to sag under eyes. The skin near the neck begins to sag.

In Europe, people are prone to skin cancer due to over exposure to the sun but this cancer is treatable. Skin cancer due to exposure to the skin is very rare in Indians.

In a nutshell, the skin protects the body against common traumas. It maintains the temperature of the body in a constant manner. It serves as a tool to excrete and make sensations. It synthesizes vitamin D required for the maintenance of the body in the presence of sunlight.

SKIN ALLERGY, BACTERIA AND LESIONS

We do get eruptions on the skin but a little care in the initial stage can save us from serious skin problems. As a matter of fact, we should not consider any eruption useless or not worthy of care. One cannot ignore as we have a number of agents that cause these eruptions; maybe those are due to mechanical irritation, parasites or germs, or even the result of some disorder of the internal organ.

Such disorders of the skin due to internal disturbance cannot be ignored because in the long run the skin disorders become the forerunner of some serious illness of the system. A person who is not well acquainted with such diseases should always consult competent doctor so that the skin ailment does not turn ugly or serious.

In the preceding chapter we have read about the structure of skin. So far we have known about the texture of skin and its diseases in the forms of lesions. Now we shall discuss about the allergic conditions of the skin, bacteriology, and lesions. It is very pertinent to discuss about these ailments in the light of homoeopathy because homoeopathy believes that all the eruptions on the skin are not particularly due to allergy, bacteria, or lesions. Is it not strange that homoeopathy believes in another angle of thinking? Homoeopathy believes that all these are outcome of some inner-body disorders and diseases.

The man who discovered Homoeopathy, Dr Hahnemann was of the opinion that all skin infections were due to some invisible live organisms that had some incubation period and could be contagious too. He had no microscope at that time yet all this was his observation. To make sure that his observations go true, he named his theory as 'theory of symptoms'. He stated miasm as an effect of microorganism on the vital force and these effect or its symptoms get transmitted to following generations.

The body has to show some symptoms when in a state of disorders or diseases and for this the skin is one of the best mediums. We shall not discuss other causes here. He classified those symptoms into three groups. All skin diseases, according to him, were due to psora, sycosis and syphilis. He named these categories of skin diseases as— Miasms.

Psora

This belongs to diseases that show itching on the skin. Along with itching, there maybe sensations like tickling, heat, cold and crawling. The skin under psora is normally dry and rough. There are no discharges and if they exist, they are scanty. If we compare the modern terminology of medical science, we can compare psora skin symptoms of lesions with irritation and inflammation of skin and also diseases connected with hypersensitive skin.

Sycosis

When Sycosis occurs the skin develops thick scales, dark discoloration, warts, moles, naevi, or abnormal hair growth. In the modern language, sycosis means indurations and overgrowths on the skin with pains.

Syphilis

Syphilis denotes the skin problems with degenerations, ulcerations and granulations. In all the symptoms of skin, there will be discharges and they are fowl smelling and their appearance is generally ugly.

They are red, coppery or brownish. The eruptions have either no sensations of pains and itching or severe pains during nights.

Besides the above three categories of skin diseases, great Hahnemann made another category of mixed Miasms. I shall not go into details of these miasms. A short introduction is sufficient for you to understand. We revert to our topic of allergies etc.

ALLERGY

An allergy is an improperly understood biological reaction which is associated with some skin diseases. Most of the times, they are their precursors. According to one school of opinion, the factors responsible for the development of immunity are interesting than the histopathological changes attached with allergy.

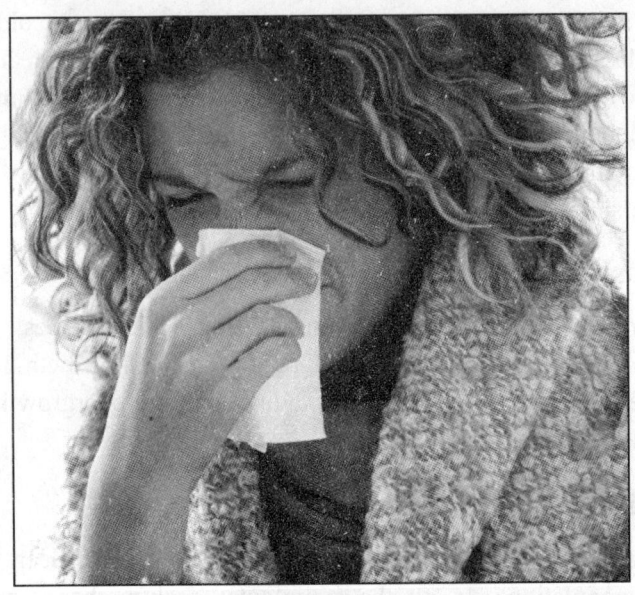

Allergy

Allergy is 'difference of reaction'. If you look at its meaning literally. It is somewhat strange that a thing which causes allergy to one subject does not cause allergy for another. The changed capacity of a tissue to react to a substance, with which it comes in touch, is an individual idiosyncrasy or peculiarity and the reaction is specific for the contact substance. This specificity is well defined as already said that an allergic item to one may not be allergic to the other.

The reaction has some identified general characteristics like inflammation, exudative in type, explosive on its on-set, and there is always a latent period between the reaction–tissue and the substance reacting. In most of the case, the changes on the skin are urticarial or eczemous. These skin diseases are typical processes of allergies.

The list of substances reacting to many persons is actually endless. A great variety of substances cause allergic cutaneous reactions. When the allergy is present, there is no pharmacological action and its effects bear no relation to the concentration in which it comes into contact with the tissue. The effects depend upon the reactivity of the tissue. A suitable reactive tissue is an exception, which maybe acquired or a congenital property of the tissue.

If a person has been eating, say cheese, for years and suddenly one fine morning he finds his skin troublesome having urticaria, such altered reactions are specific for a substance and are not due to general and non-specific cutaneous hypersensitivity. (The adjective cutaneous literally means 'of the skin' from Latin word cutis, skin).

Nowadays, it is possible to identify the substance to which the skin is allergic with the help of some chemical tests. Even if the previous contact of allergy is known, there maybe an allergy again from a substance totally new to the body. It occurs often. Under such circumstances, it has been postulated that an unknown previous contact must have occurred without major eruptions. So characteristic is this particular type of reaction of tissues that diseases conforming to it, are now identified as 'allergic' although when the contact substance with the tissue cannot be demonstrated.

It is always an assumption. In some cases, the allergy has been hereditary, so that the disease processes, which result from it, are often familial. This familial type of allergy is known as Atopy. The diseases that have been classed as atopic are hey fever, urticaria, asthma and eczema. Every case of this classification is not familial but in the presence of family history, the disease and the family affected are classed as atopic.

One should not forget the interlink of cutaneous allergy with that of 'immunity phenomena'. It is not only for skin diseases but also for other diseases of the organs and general intoxication. This is clearly demonstrated in the vaccination for smallpox etc. In all these reactions, the skin is used as index of immunity. The organ, therefore, plays an important part in the actual immunity processes since the vaccination in the skin.

Allergy is a deceptive disease not understood by definitions only and is a difficult subject to grasp. Only practical and illustrative examples can define it clearly. In the case of steatites, our subject, it is rather difficult to say that a skin disease is not due to allergic substance. Many a time, we see that some people are used to taking a lot of spices and all of a sudden, one fine morning he finds his tongue is ulcerated. He stops taking spices and the ulcers vanish. Any number of guesswork towards the causation of such an occurrence is found difficult. We have already stated that in the skin diseases, Homoeopathic treatment is our best tool since it goes by desires, aversions and modalities in the above-cited case of taking chillies. It is to be noted that we are proceeding towards knowledge while reading all this and not comparing with Homoeopathic mode of treatment at present.

BACTERIOLOGY

Bacteriology is the study of bacteria that causes disease. Louis Pasteur made the invention of bacteria and Robert Koch followed it. Bacteria may cause diseases. They are abundant in the air, the soil and the water but they are all harmless to humans though some of them cause disease and are known as pathogens. They are classified on the basis of shape—cocci (spherical) bacilli (rod shaped) and spirilla (spiral shaped).

Cocci causes pneumonia, tonsillitis, meningitis and skin affections. Bacilli causes leprosy, tuberculosis, dysentery, typhoid, and whooping cough. Spirilla cause yews, syphilis, and leptospirosis. Bacteria reproduce by dividing into two cells, which in turn divide and so on. This division can take place every twenty minutes. It produces poisons which are harmful for the human body. There are about 1600 species of bacteria and its size is measured and expressed in micrometer. These measure 0.5 to 1.2 micromillimetre in diameter.

Our normal skin has many varieties of germs and at least one parasite on its surface. Most of the time they do not cause any disease or seldom they do cause some. These germs are purely pathogenic and spread widely. They are protected always by our skin's oily or waxy surface and they are present in the orifice of sebaceous and sweat glands. They render the sterilization of the skin's surface, which is a difficult and an uncertain procedure. We can say that these are normal inhabitants of the skin but when the skin is diseased or the body is diseased, there is much wider variety of bacteria and animal parasites found on the skin. Bacteria on the skin have various stains of streptococcus, bacillus coli, yeasts and other parasites but to our naked eye, our skin appears to be clean and normal.

CLASSIFICATION OF LESIONS

Before we come to 'problem' skin and its journey to 'perfect' skin, we have to know what are skin lesions. Skin lesions are grouped in two categories—Primary skin lesions and secondary skin lesions.

Primary skin lesions are those that change the texture or colour of skin during the time of birth. Moles and birthmarks are examples of these lesions. These lesions are also acquired ones as in the case of infectious diseases, allergic reactions and environmental effects. In the case of infectious diseases some of the most common ones like acne, warts, corns or psoriasis etc., the contact dermatitis or hives are the allergic reactions and the environmental effects give rise to sunburns, pressure or extreme temperatures.

Secondary skin lesions are the after effects of primary or we can say that the changes in the skin resulting from primary skin lesions. Changes maybe normal or due to mechanical reasons, which is due to irritation or itching, the person having it scratches it. It is an outward trauma. But there is an exception to this cause too. When due to some disease in the body, there are structural changes in the skin they are also secondary lesions. Crusts, scales, fissures, scars and gangrene are the examples of secondary lesions. We shall discuss the same in the following text while differentiating both the lesions.

Primary Lesions

Erythema

Erythema can be termed as an active dilatation of the cutaneous vessels. It can be said to be the basis of all inflammatory diseases in general. The dilatation is limited to the minute capillaries in the upper most part of dermis where the redness is sharply purulent in the centre. It appears as a small red papule. If the dilatation is extended to arterioles, the redness takes the form of a flare with an ill-defined irregular margin fading into the surrounding normal skin.

Macule

Macule is nothing but discoloration of the skin either pigmentary or erythematous. Pigmentary is slightly raised above the skin and is less than a centimeter in diameter. The eruption of measles is an example of macular erythema whereas freckles can be declared as pigmentary macules.

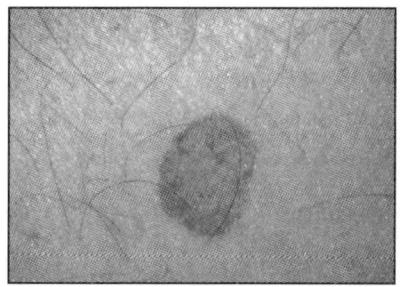

Macule

Wheal

Wheal can be called as a special development of erythema. It has various sizes and forms from a centimetre in diameter to a plaque many centimetres in surface area. It has a whitish centre with red surrounded

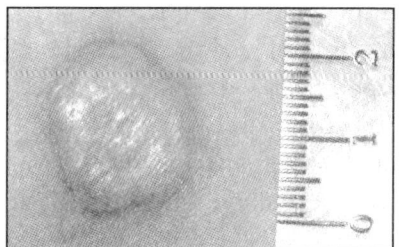

Wheal

and elevated area with a superficial lumpy feel. Dilatation and increased permeability of the capillaries and an arteriolar dilatation bring it about. It is plasma, which passes into upper dermis, makes it swell and the central lesion capillaries collapse due to pressure. The capillaries and arterioles shrink after some time and edema is reabsorbed and the whole process is over in a few hours or even less.

Papule

In comparison with wheal, papule is more a permanent lesion because in it is cellular and evolution structural changes in addition to vascular changes. These changes take time to develop and regress. It is a fluid-less inflammatory projection varying in size from a pinhead to half a centimtre in diameter and the epidermis is usually thickened. On palpitation, it may have a rubber-like feeling. Papules generally persist for a few days but they may last for weeks or even months. Lichen planus is an example of papule.

Vesicle

The vesicle is a pin-head sized elevation on the skin containing fluid. If this type of eruption with fluid is of larger size, it is called Bulla. There is not much of a difference or distinction between vesicle and bulla except that of the size. Each develops in

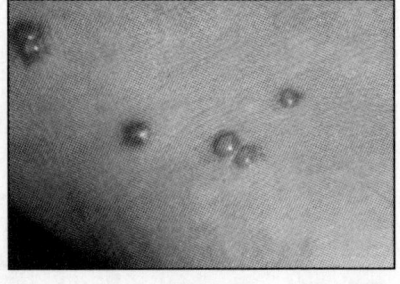

Vesicle

a characteristic fashion. A vesicle comes up by inter-epidermal edema pushing aside the cells so that small pockets of fluid are formed. These cells making the walls of the pockets undergo whitish swelling, get detached and float in the fluid.

In eczema, the vesicles are formed in this way. Both vesicles and bulla are situated high up in the epidermis (impetigo), in the middle epidermis (eczema, herpes simplex) or in the lower dermis (herpes zoster, vericella). It is upon the situation on the dermis that vesicles and bulla either rupture or dry up to form epidermic crusts. It is also common that the fluid contained in the vesicle to become turbid after a day or two as a result of pyogenic infection. In such a situation the vesicle becomes a pustule.

Pustule

It is a lesion which starts as a papule and after a few days becomes filled with pus in the centre. The centre ruptures and thick pus is discharged. Pustule generally develops at the hair follicles. Superficial pustules are located in the epidermis at the origin of a follicle and postulation may enlarge or extend to the sides of a hair follicle thus including the hair root and the sebaceous gland. Such deep-seated lesions are called Furuncles and once they are formed, they continue for a longer time. After a few weeks, they form necrosis of follicle, which is discharged in the pus as a core and healing takes place with scar-formation. In case more than two to three such follicles are affected, a plaque is formed which discharges pus at several points. Healing of such a lesion takes a lot of time and this condition is called Carbuncle.

Nodule

The nodule is exclusively a dormice lesion. It may develop as big as a pea. If it is bigger than even a pea, it is known as a Tumour, of course it should be neoplastic in nature, but if it is inflammatory in character, it is called Gumma. The nodule, tumour or a gumma has a firm deep seated cutaneous swelling and is made up of chronic type of inflammatory infiltrates like lymphocytes, epithelioid cells etc.

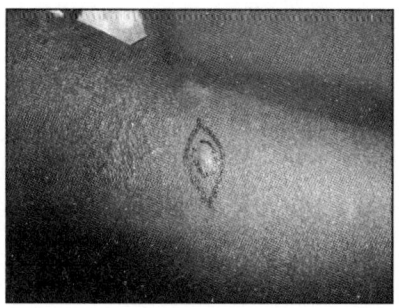

Nodule

Telangiectasia

These are very small and dilated blood vessels. They mostly appear very close to the surface of the skin. They look like tiny red boils but they denote the symptoms of disease like rosacea or scleroderma.

Secondary Lesions

As said earlier the secondary lesions are the result of mechanical scratching but scratching is not the only cause of secondary lesions. When there are structural changes in the skin due to some disease in the body, the secondary lesions also take place.

Scales

Intra-epidermal edema makes the scaling by its interference with the normal changes, which occur in the structure and chemistry of the cells when they pass from base to the surface layer. This process is called 'parakeratosis' and its cells adhere to one another to form groups on the surface, which to the naked eye appear as scales.

Secondly, when there is a rupture of vesicles or bulla, it leaves a ring of epidermal tags, which adhere to the skin in periphery but free towards the centre. These are also classed as scales. They form so quickly that parakeratosis has no time to appear on the roof of already formed scales. Scaling is common in all inflammatory cutaneous lesions and when they reach their highest peak that is, scaling over scaling, they develop and classed as 'psoriasis.' Psoriasis also comes up in non-inflammatory diseases when having nutritional disorders and also in the congenital structural abnormality known as ichthyosis. Psoriasis is one of the disease of the present era. It has red, scaly patches that are caused by epidermal cells being formed which do not reach maturity and are then discarded. The medical science has not been able to establish the exact cause of psoriasis. Shingles is another disease of the skin that needs a brief introduction. Chicken pox virus causes this and it comes as pain that turns into blisters mostly in the trunk area of the body. Similarly, another virus disease is Herpes zoster.

Crusts

Impetigo is the best example of crust. Crust is produced by coagulation and desiccation of serous and plasma exudates. In coagulation, epidermal cells are scattered and a large number of leucocytes according to stage of secondary pyogenic infection become primary exudative lesion. Superficial cellular infiltrates sometimes dry up to form crusts, as in the case of furuncles and pustules.

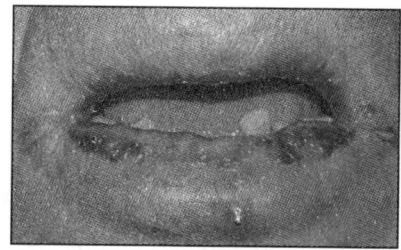
Crusts

Fissures

A mechanical splitting of the epidermis in a natural surface furrow or at the depth of a natural skin fold or a rapid scratching of skin on an inflamed area bring in fissures. They cause bleeding if they penetrate dermis. They are difficult to heal and are painful. They may appear anywhere on the body if scratching is the cause but they are commonly located behind the ears, on the knuckles, at the angles of mouth, in the groins and the natal folds.

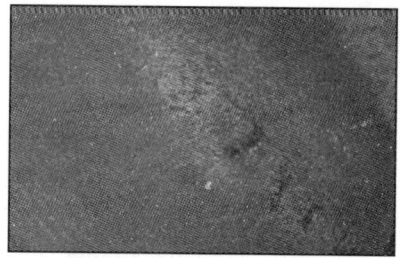
Fissures

Ulcer

The ulcer has a multiple origin. It can be by an outside trauma, necrosis of the base of a vesicle or a bulla, by sloughing to the shape of furuncle. It maybe caused by the stoppage of blood supply to an area of the skin due to spontaneous cutaneous hemorrhage or by pressure effect of tumours involving the dermis. The reasons are different but the decision to find out the actual cause of ulcer, one has to see the type of lesion that has proceeded and responsible for the loss of surface tissue by the base, shape and surroundings of the ulcer.

Scars

Scars are produced as a result of an ulcerative process besides that they are a product of injuries and trauma. It is also in some chronic inflammations in which the infiltrates of lymphocytes slowly get replaced by fibrous scar tissues and make an appearance of scar without the continuity of the surface even been broken by trauma etc.

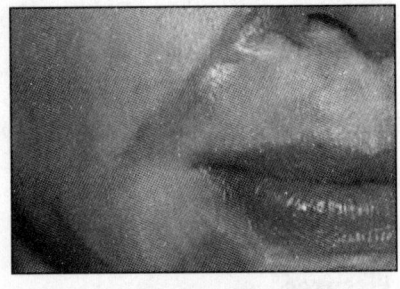

Scars

Such a condition is generally seen in the skin disease like lupus erythematosus and in scleroderma, both a press of atrophy. A scar tissue does not have hair follicles or sweat glands. It has reduced blood supply and contains no elastic fibers and no dermic papillae. It has a smooth white surface over which the natural furrows have been lost. The skin just nearby the scar maybe pigmented either temporarily or permanently. It is seen in syphilis. A thick and raised scar is called a keloid.

Gangrene

Death with putrefaction of microscopic parts of the tissue is a condition that generally can be called Gangrene. A gangrene condition lacks pulsation, venous return, and capillary response to pressure, sensation, warmth, and function. The colour of the part of the skin affected changes to purple dusky gray or brown black according to the condition of the organ of the body it has attacked. Noma and cancrum oris are its other forms while it is connected with gangrenous steatites.

Erosion

Due to some reason, when there is a loss of the epidermis, it is called erosion. It is generally a loss of hard dental tissues along the gingival margins of teeth. The lesions are shaped like dish, wedge or crescent. They generally develop on buccal surface and have sharp margins. They present hard, polished, and shiny base. The cause of erosion is not known and there is no known treatment for erosion.

Excoriation

It is a hollow crusted area that comes up due to picking at or scratching the primary lesions.

Lichenification

When the epidermis skin gets rough and hard, it is termed as lichenification. This is often a characteristic of scratch dermatitis (inflammation) and atopic dermatitis.

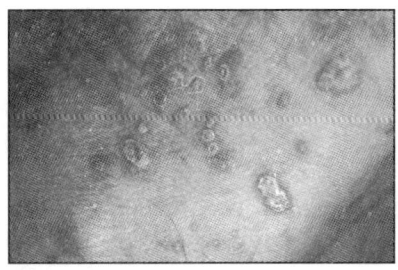
Lichenification

Atrophy (thin and wrinkled skin)

When the skin becomes thin and wrinkled, the area of that skin is called atrophy. People who use strong drugs like corticosteroids and those who get prematurely old due to some other disease are generally prone to atrophy of skin.

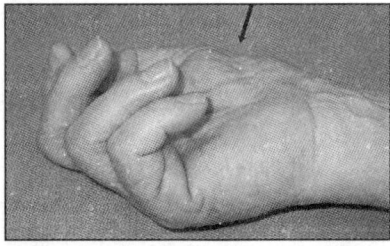
Atrophy

The doctor in case of primary or secondary lesions, has to judge whether it is a skin disorder, a trauma, a recurrent problem, or a chronic case. The heredity factor also plays a part in these lesions. The pattern of distribution also has to be observed. Skin disorders also create many psychological problems, which have to be examined by the doctor. In such cases, Homoeopathy has been long known to be very effective.

CLASSIFICATION OF PRIMARY AND SECONDARY LESIONS

The classification of primary and secondary lesions is made here to make an assessment for doctors and students of homoeopathy.

Acne

Acne is found mostly in young girls having oily skin.

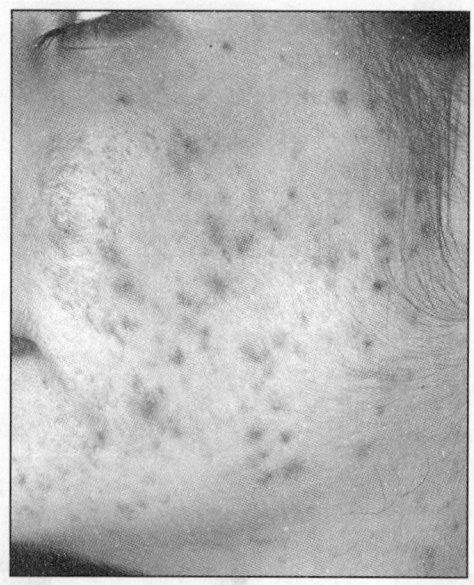

Acne

Fungal Skin Infections

Ringworms

Tinea versicolor Candidiasis

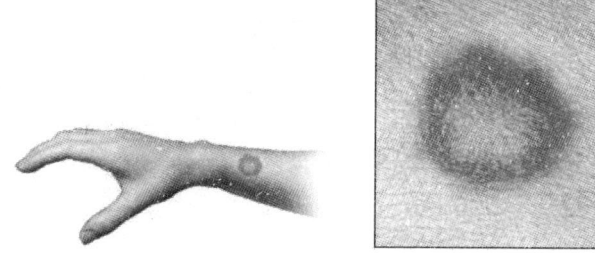

Fungal skin infection

Blisters

Dermatitis herpetifornis

Bullous Pemphigoid Pemphigus

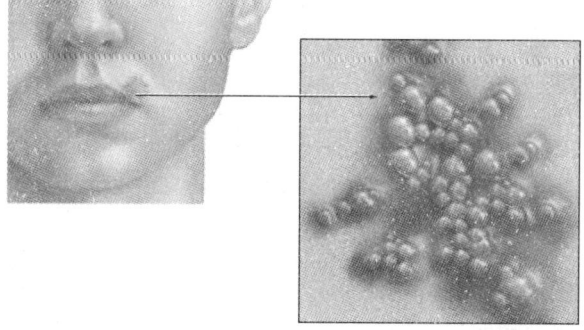

Blisters

Bacterial Infections

- Erythrasma
- Cellulitis
- Folliculitis

- Abscesses
- Carbuncles
- Impetigo
- Necrotizing skin disorders

Scales

Skin growths (non-cancerous)

- Cysts
- Fibroids
- Keloids
- Lipomas
- Moles
- Seborrhoeic Keratoses
- Skin tags
- Dermatofibromas

Disorders Pigmentation

- Albinism
- Melasma
- Vitiligo

Viral Infections

- Warts
- Molluscum Contagiosum

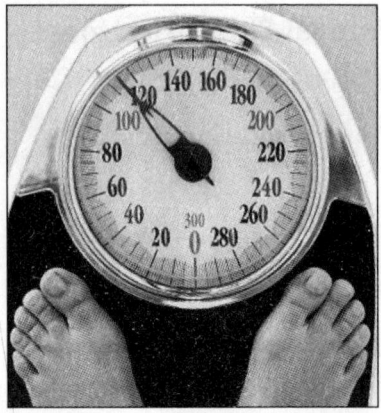
Scales

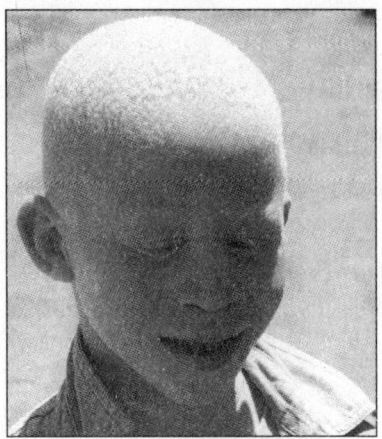
Albinism

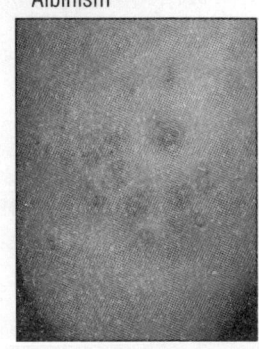
Warts

Rashes and Itching

- Rashes due to drugs taking
- Dermititis
- Itching

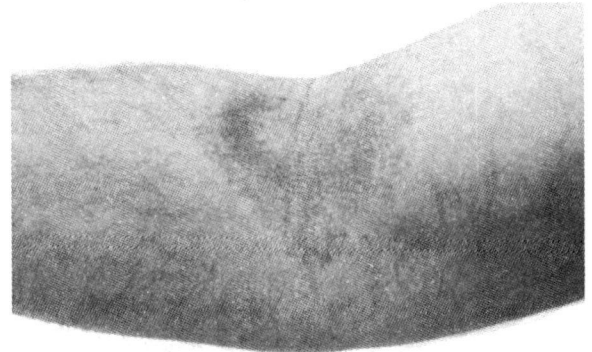

Rashes and itching

- Lichen planus
- Keratosis pilaris
- Erythema Multiforme and Nodusum
- Granuloma
- Psoriasis
- Rosacea

Chapter 3

Examining Skin Conditions, Texture and Health

DIFFERENCE BETWEEN SKIN-DISEASES AND SKIN-DISORDERS

Before we enter into the subject of the book we have to know that skin disorders and skin diseases are two different aspects. It will be even better if we know who has a healthy body with a healthy skin.

If we break up the word disease, it will be 'dis' and 'ease', which means when the body is not at ease. To make it more clear, health is order and disease is disorder. This is one aspect of understanding. There is another explanation. 'Dis' means deprived of and 'ease' means comfort. Comfort here means health. When one is deprived of health and its comfort, it is a disease. The uneasiness or discomfort is because there is some infection, viral or bacteria that has affected the body and the body is not feeling at ease.

Disorder is something that is never welcome. It is either voluntarily invited by the person or maybe the result of circumstances. If someone has taken the food that is not agreeable to him, the food is bound to cause discomfort and could lead to skin allergy, diarrhoea, flatulence (gas), dyspepsia or constipation.

Similarly, an exposure to extreme cold winds or hot winds could lead to sunlight allergy or cold-frost, colds, or fevers. Skin allergy, sneezing, cold, and cough could be caused by over drenching of the body. If these maladies are treated in time, they are cured soon. All these are called disorders.

It is a universal fact that disorders can get converted to diseases if not taken care of at the right time. The internal- self of the body is constantly reacting to the external environments. The disorder of the body takes place when these two internal and external are thrown out of balance.

Disease can be classified in reference with its site of manifestation, which maybe in the skin, lungs, liver, heart, and so on. Disease has to be associated with some cause. Diseases have their origin in three ways—physical, psychological and spiritual. If it is physical, it has many methods to get eliminated. If it has psychological reasons, the treatment becomes difficult and takes long to cure but if it is of spiritual nature, it is not possible to cure any disease. Spiritual stands for 'negative thinking' here.

PARAMETERS OF SKIN DISORDERS AND DISEASES

Since ages, skin diseases have been in existence and doctors have been dealing with them through various therapies. Earlier the outlook of skin diseases and disorders were different and today the treatment to cure them is completely different.

Earlier, the skin diseases were treated with the help of leaves of plants. The burning and banding of the site of infection, use of leeches to suck blood from the diseased part and applying various kinds of ointments that were made on 'hear and say' method was in practice to heal the skin diseases. Today, the methods of treatment have changed and proven ointments or medicines are given to the patient after making proper diagnosis.

According to Dr J.C. Burnett, skin is an integral living organ of the body and it has a definite relation with the internal health of the body. Healthy skin can never exist without the existence of internal health. Of course, exceptions do exist. Skin disease can appear without the disturbance of internal health of a body as well. It may occur due to external traumas.

According to the science of biology, the longevity of skin is fed from internal resources and the diseases are also the outcome of the deranged internal condition of the body. Skin diseases are, therefore, not organic but can be due to constitutional causes.

According to the principles of Homoeopathy, all skin diseases have relations with the health of one's internal organs. Mental and emotional disturbance also play an important role in bringing about skin diseases. The skin is connected with all the internal organs of the body and health is a state of complete physical, mental, and social well-being, not merely the absence of disease.

Every person has a health condition typical to his body. The daily activities and behaviour of a person's family and their members promote, protect, or damage the health depending upon their lifestyle. This is the reason why some people have good health due to good upkeep that include the diet, family atmosphere, temperament and behaviour to deal with domestic problems, console each other and live peacefully.

Any change in health will surely make a good or bad impact on the skin. There is no doubt about this theory as skin is a fibro-elastic membrane that maybe truly called the envelope of the human body. If the contents of this envelope (body health inside) get rotten or decomposed, the envelope (skin) will surely show marks of decay. This truth is vice versa. If the envelope (skin) faces harsh environment, extremities of climate, or traumas, the contents of envelope will get the affected.

It is beyond doubt that every person has different health condition and variable skin diseases. What are those parameters that make health and skin diseases variable? Here are some conditions which vary from each person to the other. They are:-

- Heredity
- Constitution
- Environment
- Profession
- Gender
- Race
- Stress and depression
- Mood
- Climate
- Traumas
- Food
- Drugs
- Sex

These are direct causes but there are local causative factors in idiopathic diseases that are influenced by underlying conditions of organic substances. It is difficult to relate the general underlying idiopathic condition of a body with symptomatic appearance on the skin (cutaneous) but we have made these notions especially based on homoeopathic theory that every skin disease is the outcome of some internal malady.

Talking of heredity, mention maybe made of diseases like syphilis and ichthysis or even psoriasis/eczema. Actually it depends upon the race and nation to which one belongs. Many countries are prone to dermatitis, keloids, and other skin diseases. Age and sex also plays a part in certain skin conditions.

Diseases like tuberculosis, scrofulous or strumous diathesis could trigger the development of these diseases due to constitutionals effects. Eruptive fevers and syphilis are also of the same causation of constitution. Such maladies often appear in the middle or even at old age. Diabetes, Asthma, and certain cardiac diseases also come under the same causation of constitutional and heredity effects.

The causative factors for skin disease are seasons or climate as well. We know that the outcome of urticaria, itching, intertrigo or miliria are also result of hot season whereas cold season has pruritis, chilblains, frostbites, triggering of existing eczema or psoriasis.

Similarly, personal hygiene plays a vital role in aggravating the skin diseases. Unclean or filthy habits may lead to diseases of the skin.

Under professional causation factor, those who work or deal in chemical factories or do manual work in factories preparing acids, dyes, bricks, iron moulds, X-ray clinics, dealers of alkalis or potash may experience an aggravation of their existing skin diseases or even get skin diseases that were not earlier not there.

Menstruation has also has an important relation with skin diseases. If a skin disease exists, the onset of menses (before or after menses) may aggravate the skin diseases.

Similar is the case with pregnancy, lactation and menopause. Ingestion of some drugs in small or large doses can produce many elementary eruptions on the skin. Of course some people are prone to them and not all of us. This is a phenomenon which is completely personal and typical to different individuals.

On our skin there are erotogenic zones that have properties of stimulation. These zones are full of sensitivities for sexual acts. Those who have pruritis (itch) of vulva or anuses have a tendency to rub to satisfy their libido. Such rubbing or scratching can initiate pains but these are perverted pleasures. Such acts generate guilty feelings. (Rubbing or scratching penis or vulva that is masturbation). And as a result there erupts skin diseases like allergic eczema, hives, ace etc. I have given some of the factors that lead to skin diseases and not all including parasites, scratching, contagions and cutaneous irritants.

One aspect here is common to all cases of skin diseases is that in each causation factor, it is the internal health condition of the body that has triggered the skin ailments. Factors like food, diet, mood, stress, and worries mentioned above shall be discussed later in this book.

WHO POSSESSES HEALTHY SKIN?

In our society there are many people who are compelled to get up early in the morning because they have to attend morning shift in their factories or reach office in time because the office is far away and it takes a long time to reach there. Many people have to get up early to see that their children reach school in time dressed properly along with their packed lunch. There are people, mostly in northern India, who get up early in the morning because they have to fetch fresh milk for the household use. These people take a lot of care to see the milkman milking the cow or the buffalo and hence reach the place of milkman early in the morning. In other words, the nature of work makes all of these people get up early in the morning. The moral of all this is that such people who go out into the nature early in the morning get fresh air and do some walking do not fall ill soon and maintain good healthy skin.

Now there are also people who do not get up early in the morning but have a definite routine of work, which the above mentioned category is not accustomed to. Such people take care that they clean their teeth, have regular baths, do a little exercise at home, take selective nutritional diet, do lot of walking to purchase domestic goods, avoid the usage of cars or scooters and are ready to help others in the times of need. These persons have a fixed schedule and never forget to exercise at home. Such people also maintain good healthy skin.

If the routine of both the above types of people continues, the skin diseases do not attack them soon. But disorders may eventually be caused by exposures to allergens or some errors in diet.

STRUCTURAL DIFFERENCE AND SKIN DISEASES

In the very first place think how do you see and judge your personality? Just stand before a mirror and watch you body. Do you like it? Is it proportionate with all curves in right places? Are you pleased with your complexion or the colour? Do you want to present your body image to the people in the way it looks or do you want to improve its image for the people to like? This is the image of your body that brings in you the confidence and you develop a sense of self-liking. This is possible only when you keep your body fit and make it presentable in appearance to others. It is the exercise and good diet that can fulfill your dream of a good skin and an attractive body. This is one aspect concerning your outward or physiological looks.

There is another aspect of looking at your body. Most of the times it is by the structure of your body by which you might be remembered by your friends nd relatives. People would remember you by the structure of your body first in case they do not know your name. They would say the man or woman in question was lean, thin, fat, round, short or long and so one. The police identify the criminals by the description of their structure and not personality. This is called structural appearance.

STRUCTURAL DIFFERENCES AND NATURE OF SKIN

Skin can be divided into three categories on the basis of their structure. They are lean (ectomorph), rounded, (endomorph) and muscular (mesomorph).

If you are lean, thin and belong to ectomorph, it would be difficult for you to develop a muscular body even if you took efforts regarding your diet and exercise. I said difficult but not impossible. Ectomorph people can also develop muscular body but it requires great effort and training from professional gym experts. Your contribution to the industry of beauty products is lesser than endomorphs.

Now suppose that you are an endomorph, then you will be liable to keep growing fat and keep gaining weight because of heredity reasons. Parts of your body like your thighs, stomach and buttocks may have excessive fat than is required. Here again, it is difficult to get a muscular body without special efforts under the guidance of a professional. You are actually helping the skin-care industry to grow and flourish. You not only try exercise routines but also use beauty supplements to a greater extent.

If you are mesomorph, you are lucky because you already possess a muscular body by the dint of the genetic order. You also have enough stamina. What you need is a regular maintenance exercise routine and a balanced diet to maintain what God has given you. If you possess a dark or a dusty complexion and need a fair one, all your attempts would go waste and you would have to remain what you are.

Irrespective of the structural differences of the skin (lean, rounded or fat) the skin can have disorders and diseases. Generally, there is some relation of structural difference and skin diseases. Fat persons sweat more and get tired easily when exerting and are prone to oily skin. Please take a note that these rules are only suggestive of the consequences of structural differences of a person and may not be taken guaranteed.

Chapter 4

Common Avoidable Problems of the Skin

COMMON AVOIDABLE PROBLEMS

Our skin undergoes many types of changes based on various conditions like health, climate, diet and life style as we have already discussed. The beauty of this change is that some changes are for the betterment of the skin whereas some changes do not favour the skin and turn into diseases. If one is particular in observing the condition of the skin, he or she can easily deal with the problems. Here, we shall discuss how problem skin can change to perfect skin and perfect skin can change to problem skin.

If we go on to define a problem, it maybe said that a problem is something that is difficult to deal with. Similarly, if we try to define perfection, we may say that it is a condition devoid of any problem, complete and flawless. We all know that skin is accustomed with hazards of our environment. It has to face traumas, frictions, bruises, heat, cold, harsh winds, storms, rains, light and all these impacts bring in lesions on the skin. Even if one is free of these factors, which is impossible, one is adept to genetically influenced disorders. No one has a perfect skin or a flawless skin. You may find the face of a person glowing with health with no problem in the skin according to the age but there maybe some abnormalities on the skin other than the face. When you see a person with sound health and a charming face without any eruptions, it comes under the category of perfect skin. The word 'perfect' used in this book means sound and glowing with health. Problem skin to perfect skin is a journey of knowledge that is to know more about the problem skin and the ways of how to make it perfect.

The effect of sunlight

Today, all of us know that sunlight or the solar radiation has an impact on the human body. Our skin is capable of protecting itself from excessive sunlight and ultraviolet rays. The outer layer or the epidermis of our skin absorbs some of the heat and

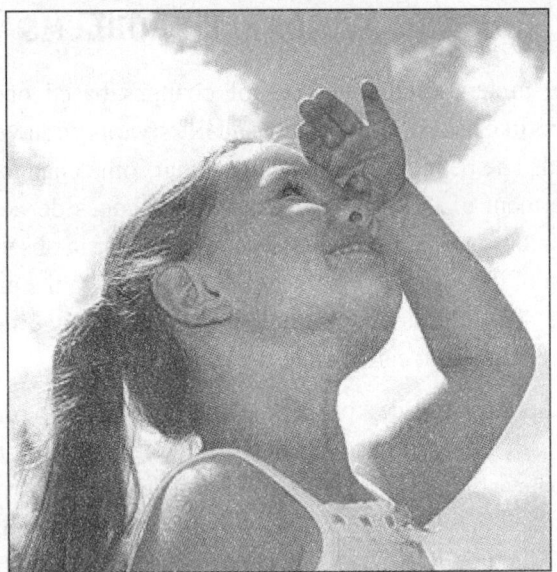

The effect of sunlight

the melanin pigment of the skin further saves whatever is not protected by epidermis. If one remains in the sunlight for quite a longer time, there will be acute sunburns turning the skin red and black. After few days when the exposure to sun will be discontinued, the skin will return to its original complexion.

Those who live in the deserts or in villages are acclimatized to the sunlight. So, they do not develop any sort of itching, scales or other diseases except the permanent tan on the skin that is exposed to the sunlight. Generally the face, forehead, nose, and cheeks are affected and there is a change in colour.

Many of us must have seen people wearing bare minimum clothes that is only under garments and working in the sun. Such people develop a different kind of tan on the body on the exposed parts leaving the covered parts of the body possessing the actual skin colour. The same can be seen in the case of ladies. Their exposed parts like face, neck, arms etc. are discoloured due to sunlight and the covered parts retain the original colour of the skin. In the months of winter, this discoloration of exposed skin wears out. This is the best example where skin with a problem becomes perfect without the use of medicines.

Frost Bite

It is quite a known fact that while the heat expands the skin, the cold contracts the skin. People living at high altitudes experience this particular disease called frostbite. Our defense personnels working at high altitudes also become victims of frostbite when their body parts are exposed to harsh, strong and cold winds even for few minutes. Most of the times the hands, feet, toes, fingers, ears, nose and cheeks become red, swollen, numb, and white. If the bite is mild and the exposure has not been too much, simple treatment of heating (mild heating) the affected body parts and bringing the patient to moderate climate brings back the normal condition of the skin. Initially heating may bring in some swelling of the parts but it becomes normal later. It is noteworthy that when the skin was not exposed to the strong cold winds, it was quite perfect and when it was exposed, it gradually changed to problem skin. On warming the problem skin, it became perfect again. This is perhaps the best natural example of a journey from problem to perfect skin. Chilblains are different from frostbite and need medical attendance.

Shoe-blisters

Many a time when we wear very tight shoes, the impact is on the outer lining of the skin the epidermis. There occurs considerable friction between the skin and the shoe. This friction produces blisters. Not going into the details of how these are formed let me give you the simplest solution. The simplest solution to this problem is to avoid using those tight shoes with which the blisters occured. Within two or three days, the blisters will be cured if there has been no complication of some other disease (diabetes) that delays healing. The skin is generally back to normal and the feet becomes perfect.

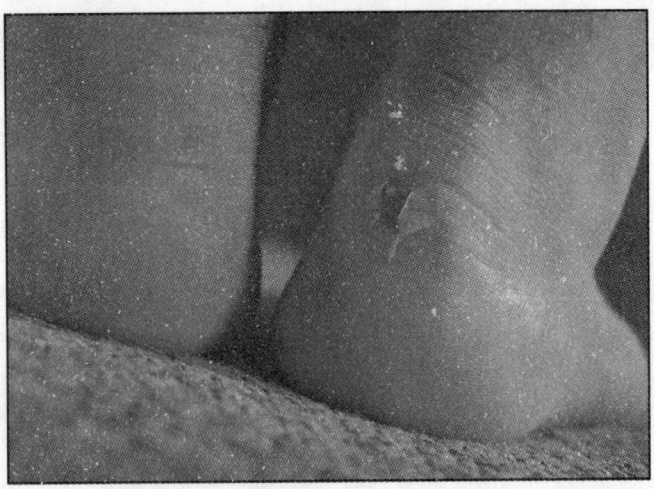

Shoe-blisters

In this case, the practical approach to bring the problem skin to perfect skin is to oil the new shoe at the place where it has bitten or pinched. The second best option is to replace the shoe. Application of some anti-infection cream or even coconut oil will serve the purpose too. It is better to avoid excessive wetting of the affected area and take homoeopathic medicine like Allium cepa under the guidance of a doctor.

CORNS

Corns is a term is well-known to people although it has medical complications and one has to go to a doctor for operation if the corns are not cured with the help of corn-plaster available at the chemist shops. Corns come under the callosities given in details below and are generally a consequence of

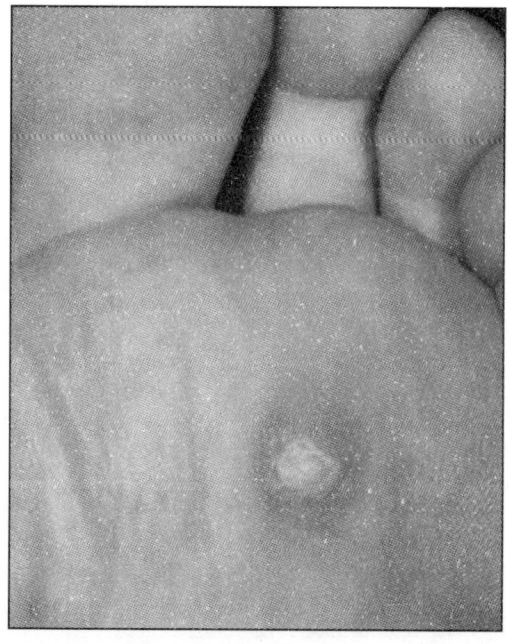

Corn

ill-fitting shoe or some projected nail in the soles inside the shoe. If this projection in the shoe is ignored and the wearer continues to wear the shoe, then there is continuous pressure created on the outer layer of the skin of soles, which in the long run travels to the second inner layer of the skin. This means it creates pressure on the nerves. It gradually becomes painful especially when the area of affection is pressed directly.

Once the corns are cured with a corn-plaster or with help of homoeopathic medicines, the skin returns to normal. Antim crud is the medicine that should be taken under the guidance of the doctor.

CALLOSITIES

People who plough in fields, conduct mason's work, lift heavy rods everyday or do any type of manual work regularly, they get callosities on their palms near finger joints or in between the

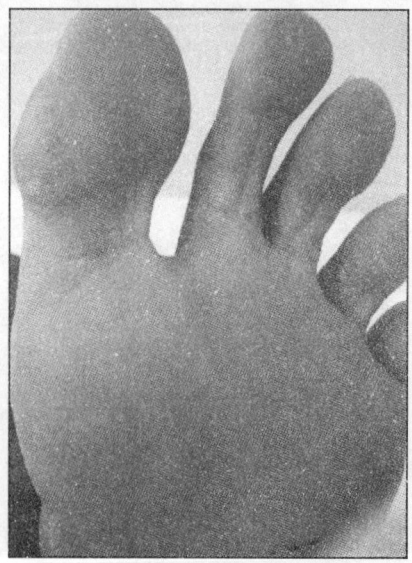

Callosities

thumb and the index finger muscles. People who walk without shoes on uneven grounds of villages and forests, those who have abnormal soles of feet or abnormal gait, they also get callosities on their soles. Even people going to offices in the cities and holding rods above the head in the buses regularly may develop soft callosities due to friction of their palm-finger joints with the iron rod. There is no remedy for such soft callosities and when the farmers, masons, labourers and office-goers stay away from their work for a considerable period of time, the callosities disappear though they are subjected to reappearance when they resume their routine work.

There is not much of pain in the locations of the callosities. Only some irritation is felt and hence the people do not bother about the callosities. Some people even show off their callosities marks to their friends saying that they have joined a gym and their hard work on bars and dumbbells have brought in the callosities.

In Homoeopathy, we have many medicines that should be taken under the guidance of doctor (Ruta, Calcarea fluorica, Graphites, Thuja and Antim crudum etc) in such. The real relief comes when the particular job that brings in callosities is discontinued for quite a number of months. Callosities are a significant example of how problematic skin can become perfect skin again.

These above-mentioned examples are cited just to tell the readers that most of the problem skin or common disorders can disappear on their own provided the individual affected is cautious and knows the trait of each disorder.

Chapter 5

Seven Factors that Balance the Beauty of Skin

Life has changed considerably all over the world today. The life of the new generation is ruled by the television, mobile phones, computers and the fast-food. Sleeping late at night and getting up late in the morning has become a normal routine for them. So, their health is just affected adversely leading to many kinds of disorders.

Some of them who can afford the cost, join gyms or exercise clubs in the hope of improving their destroyed health. The rest try various types of cosmetics to regain the lost vigour and beauty. The condition of health of a girl or a boy in the rural area is also getting a downward bent. They are also caught up in the trap laid by lotions, creams, beauty soaps and shampoos that were not known to them earlier. Earlier, the instructions of our parents paved the way to our good health which are completely neglected and as a consequence, our health is also affected. The young do not eat the diet they used to eat traditionally. Introduction of packed tins or ready made vegetables, noodles and the like have made their life easy amidst their very busy routine office. It is noteworthy that the western countries have realised that the Indian life-style and Indian diet is absolutely free of toxins. It is this Indian life style that can establish the best of skin-health. In India very few people go for plastic surgery. On the other hand, in the western countries, there is a new name given to this trend of surgery called 'Plastic Beauty'. For this purpose, many Botox clinics (plastic surgery clinics where wrinkles are erased with the help of medicinal injections) have been opened and are running very successfully. We will discuss about Botox in the forthcoming chapters.

It is worth the thought that why Europeans praise the Indian life style? It's due to our method of treating ourselves through our lifestyle. In spite of all the bad habits we are still nearer to the nature and we still have some routine in life and our diet.

Coming to skin conditions of the young and old, it is mostly gift of heredity and are a result of the regional setting, climate and the regional dietary habits. We have adopted by traditions certain food habits and these habits make a person prone to skin health or gives rise to skin disorders. A slight change in their food habits can trigger off a skin disease or make a decrease in the diseases as well. The skin conditions have a connection with the diet. A diet taken at home is the best, whatever maybe the region, or state, we live in. Make the eating habit regularly in time.

CONSTIPATION

Constipation is the disorder of inactive people who do not bother to exercise and have a sedentary lifestyle. It unfailingly leads to headaches, fatigue and bad breath besides making the complexion dull (lack of brightness). When one does not pass stool or there is infrequent bowel movement, then one feels that there is something left in the abdomen which is not clear. Such a condition is called constipation. With constipation, you will be restless, feel uneasy and may have to release gas frequently. Constipation is a serious problem which if ignored, the condition may lead to hemorrhoids (piles), which means that there is underlying intestinal disease.

Clear bowls play a vital role in maintaining the skin health or complexion one is born with. When constipated, there will be lot of metabolic changes in the body resulting in the quality of blood. It is the blood that is polluted in constipated conditions and this invites many skin diseases besides making complexion dull and devoid of lustre. No constipation means clear complexion and removal of pimples and acne etc. from face and the body.

Easy Evacuation

Drink plenty of water early in the morning after getting up without any intake of food or tea or without rinsing your mouth. It is suggested to take a minimum of two glasses full of water. This water should be stored in a copper vessel the previous night. Switch on a radio or a tape-recorder to listen to devotional songs in praise of God.

Walk

It is said that walking helps a lot Walk as much as you can around the room for a few minutes and go to the toilet. The purpose is preventing constipation, build self-confidence and enhancing mental power.

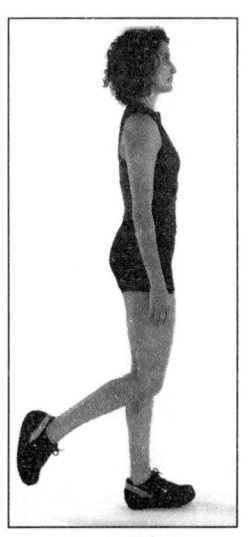
Walk

Defecate with ease without straining. You may clutch your upper and lower teeth together keeping the mouth closed and then evacuate. This will not only strengthen the roots of your teeth and gums but you will have easy evacuation. Do not strain or exert too much while evacuation. If you feel that your bowl is not moving and getting cleared, you could adopt any of the following methods.

Press thumbs of your both hands against the skin below corners of lower lip. Continue pressure count up to twenty. Release the pressure and count ten now. Repeat this act of pressing and releasing for three times.

If this method does not work, try another. Put both your hands on both feet so that the palms are pressing them. Now while you are in this pose, elevate your buttocks upwards slowly to an extent that your calves and thighs make an angle of ninety degrees or more. While elevating or raising the buttocks, take a deep breathing inside. Hold the breath for a while when your buttocks are in elevated position and then release the breathing out slowly. At the same time lower your hips to normal as you sit on feet. Repeat this act twice or thrice and you will have easy evacuation. Apart from these you may:

- Increase the intake of green vegetables and fruits having high fiber. Avoid going to hotels, taking fast food or junk food, taking fried and heavy meals.
- Take a glass of apple juice everyday day if possible.
- Start morning or evening walks with some light exercises.
- Take at least two glasses of water after you get up from bed in the morning. Take one glass of milk every night before going to sleep.
- Increase your intake of water per day.
- Take medicines suggested by Homoeopathy.
- Avoid a sedentary lifestyle. Take Nux vomica 200, two times a day for three days.
- If the stool is hard stool, dry, and you have a desire for dry food, take the homeopathy medicine called Alumina 200 (better for old people and children), in the same above manner.

- Stool hard, dry, burnt, too large, no desire, thirst more at long intervals: Bryonia 200 in the same above manner.
- Patient feels better and normal when constipated fat flabby chilly patients: Calcarea carb 30, three times a day for seven days.
- If one is constipated but can pass stool only when in the standing position, take the homeopathy medicine called Causticum 200 weekly one dose for three weeks.
- Chronic constipation of old peoples with sinking feeling in stomach, tongue flabby and white: Hydrastis-Q. Take 8 drops in half cup of water, twice daily for 7 days.
- In chilly patients, stool goes back into rectum, when partially expelled: Silicea 200, weekly one dose for three weeks.

Home Remedies for Constipation

There are many home remedies that can cure constipation but the usage of water best is. Keep half a litre of clean drinking water in a mug or a vessel made of copper. This water should be taken just after getting up from bed. Simply drinking the water is not advised. Close both the nostrils of your nose and then drink the whole of the water sitting on the bed itself. Now lie on your left side on the bed for five minutes and then get up. Walk in the room itself for some time and you will surely feel like going to the toilet for evacuation. If your constipation has existed for a very long time, go on doing this for a number of days and you will have gradual relief. Those having constipation should have high fiber diet and avoid much of refined, processed, spicy and fatty food. During a day, drink at least six to seven glasses of water or water based fluids like fruit juice. Apple and grape juice are better options. One should take light meals, take it in time, and also some milk at bedtime.

Use of Isabgol and Trifla

'Isabgol' are herbal flakes available in the market sparingly in any chemist shop. It is a very popular medication given for constipation. I have seen prescriptions of doctors of prestigious medical institutions prescribing 'Isabgol' along with the other medicines. One to two tablespoons full of Isabgol should be taken with warm some milk at night for at least 7 days and then discontinued for some days. As and when one feels constipation again, the same routine of intake can be repeated. I have tried this on my patients and found it to be very successful except in stubborn few cases where the patients are over the age of sixty years.

In case of stubborn constipation of older people, when isabgol does not work efficiently, trifla can be taken. Trifla is a powder which is the mixture of amla, Hararh and Behra, three herbs available in the market. It is manufactured by all well-known Ayurvedic medicines manufacturing companies. One teaspoonful of trifla should be taken with warm water at night. This should be taken for three days and the results will be seen. If there is improvement, take it on every alternate day for at least 15 days. Later whenever there is constipation, this can be repeated in the above manner once more.

Where the stools have not been coming for days, the best laxative is a glass of hot milk in which two teaspoons of 'ghee' are added. This should be taken at night while going to bed.

For any problems related to beauty of skin, acne, pimples, boils, it is better to get the same diagnosed by a competent doctor before going in for application of facial creams etc.

HYGIENE

Our body has three basic needs—good food, exercise and sleep. All these three basic needs have to be observed along with cleanliness otherwise they are of no use. If food is not made in clean atmosphere, if rest is not taken at a clean place and if exercise is conducted in unclean suffocating place, there may occur skin diseases and they may not leave the body till proper hygienic measures are taken. Cleanliness can be divided in two categories—personal hygiene and public hygiene.

Public Hygiene

This is an important factor to keep our body free of skin diseases. If the environment is not clean, how can the skin remain free of diseases? The first is cleaning of our house regularly so that we do not live in dirt. This includes cleaning of floors, windows and doors, changing dirty curtains, sofa covers and pillow covers, dusting the mats, chairs tables, glass-panes, the television, computer, washing machine and other gadgets in the house. Removal of cobwebs from the corners is also essential. If the spiders make a web over your bed and by chance if it falls on your skin, there will be painful rashes that will need the doctor's attention.

Areas like under the bed, sofa, chairs, and tables should be regularly cleaned. The bed on which you sleep should be cleaned daily and the bed sheets should be changed at regular intervals. During the rainy season and the and the winter, the quilts and blankets should be kept in the sun for sometime everyday if possible. Everything in the house should be kept in order and at a selected place from where they can be procured easily. All the dust and dirt or waste papers and kitchen waste should be collected in wastebaskets and handed over to the sweepers available. In case there is no arrangement, it should be taken to a place fixed by the government for depositing this waste.

The cleaning starts from home and then to the streets, locality, and finally goes on to the town. A clean house is one of the important factors that can give rise to good and healthy skin of the members of that house.

Personal Hygiene

In personal hygiene, the foremost ingredient is mental cleanliness. One has to be clean, laborious, and alert and have patience of mind. His mental make up should not have anger, perversions, greed and jealousy. Man should always believe in God. He should pray to God everyday thanking Him for giving life and its bounties. To clean the mind of a person and to gather patience, it is the prayers that help. It is the prayers that make a man strong in determination and will power.

They say that a man with a strong mind will surely have a strong body. Mental power is more valuable than physical power. The prayers should be made at a definite place and a definite time so that it becomes a routine of day. You may believe in any religion. It makes no difference because it is ONE power that rules the universe and we may call that power by different names.

The next most important thing is personal hygiene next. If our skin is cleaned regularly, there are very few chances of skin disorders. Our body needs cleaning everyday and it is our duty to keep it clean but this outer cleanliness is as important as the inner cleanliness of the body.

Our body is like a machine that runs with food and then excretes the waste matters. If a steam engine runs with coal, it has to discard the coal ash. Similarly, our body also discharges stool, urine, and sweat. If the discharges are not in order, they have the worst impact on the skin and facial setup. These discharges should be in order so that inner body does not get stagnant and the machine does get upset. Our body works with a predetermined rhythm and if this rhythm is maintained by good food intake, exercise and permissible discharges.

We have another kind of hygiene called the mental hygiene. It also relates to skin conditions. If we persistently think about negative things and evils happenings, it affects the skin condition. This is confirmed by the laws of Miasms in Homoeopathy. We shall discuss about this later in this book.

DISCHARGES OF THE BODY

Given below are the rules that are to be observed for regulating the discharges to avoid skin diseases

Stool

The timing of passing stool should be fixed. If one is going for passing the stool sometimes in the afternoon after eating, sometimes in the evening and sometimes in the night, this will be called as a bad stool habit and the person is likely to suffer from some disease. Passing stool two times a day (morning and evening) is considered ideal for cleaning the stomach. If one goes for stool even three times and the stool is normal, there is no harm. The condition is that one should feel that nothing is left in the stomach.

The toilets should be clean. They should fulfill the purpose. The Indian type of toilet seats creates direct pressure on the thighs and legs and the stomach and this pressure helps in evacuation.

Some people take newspaper or magazine with them to the toilet and say that evacuation becomes easy. It is all in the mind. If they are able to clear their stomach by reading papers, there is no harm in taking paper to the toilet. The rule is that all the attention should be towards evacuation so that nothing is left in the stomach. Such concentration cannot be there while reading.

After stool, the wiping of anus by toilet paper maybe good in the European or American countries due to cold climate but in India, it is not hygienic. Continuous wiping the outer anal area may irritate the skin and cause inflammation can occur due to sweating. Sweating in the Indian climate cannot be avoided. If there are some minute stool particles left in the anal area due to incomplete wiping by toilet paper, the sweating could spread the infection of stool and end in inflammation. The water is therefore the best medium to clean the anus after stool. There is no chance of anything remaining around the anus area.

The water used for washing the anus should never be hot. Always use cold water even in winter. Hot water has the capability of spreading the infection existing in the of remains of stool. One should not exert power to expel stool. If one strains for stool expulsion, there is chance that he will damage your the anus and the rectum. The strain is directly on the veins of the rectum that might explode because of friction of hard stool with the walls of rectum. In the long run, this habit leads to haemorrhoids. Prolapse of rectum are also due to this reason.

Urination

In a day about one and half litres of urine discharge is normal. If there is dribbling of urine, excess of urine discharge, urine is very yellow, red or milky white or comes out with pain, or there is retention of urine and bladder is distended, if the stream of urine becomes variable, weak and tends to stop and start, you should not waste time and consult the doctor at once.

In healthy condition, the urine is generally light yellow in colour. In many cases, the urine falls vertically without any force. Normally, the flow of urine should appear like an arc and not vertical. If it is not so, consult the doctor.

If one drinks a good quantity of water, the urine will be regulated in good quantity.

Do not postpone your urge for urination at any time. Postponing the urge of urine-passing exerts pressure on the bladder. The bladder has a limited space to expand beyond which, it cannot inflate. The result is that the pressure of urine and its retention in the bladder makes the walls of bladder thick, especially at the neck. This pressure is transmitted to prostate gland through urethra and compresses the gland. Compression means widening of the area of bladder but squeezing the area of opening of bladder. The prostate gland is like a ring over the urethra. This ring expands due to inflammation or increases its weight thus compressing the bladder. If the urge for urination is suppressed time and again, the prostate gland goes on expanding gradually. Do not suppress the urge to urinate.

WALKING

In the olden times, there were not adequate means of transport. Horses and carriages were used for long journeys. Later cycles were added and this is being used now also. People in those times depended mostly upon walking when the distance was not much. But now even for fetching bread or milk from a nearby market we use scooters, cars, and cycles and do not go by walking. Walking is a majestic remedy for improving the skin conditions. For young men and women, walking should not be just walking but brisk walking. Walking improves the blood circulation. There are sixty thousand blood vessels in our body. These vessels or capillaries make our flesh glow. These vessels and capillaries irrigate our skin. If we do not walk briskly, and take rest, less number of the capillaries will open.

Walking improves the state of mind and disposition. It has a tranquilizing effect and one may get fresh ideas after walking. Many problems of life are solved when the mind becomes fresh after walking. Mind has no time to think during walking and hence is fresh after the walk.

Walking removes constipation, muscles pain and low back pain. It is not essential to make a fixed time for walking. Walking can be done at any time, morning, or evening or even after dinner. You can even walk from your house to the bus stand. It will only bring you back to your original shape.

If one follows the above precautions, one would be less prone to skin diseases.

SLEEP AND REST

In order to maintain good skin health, sleep and rest are very essential. You can yourself experience the condition of your health when you do not get sleep due to some ceremony, celebration or any other reason. Whole of the day you would be restless and would feel weak. Your skin would be burning or would be cold and you would be feeling discomfort all through your skin. Even if you try to sleep in the daytime, you will not get the comfort which is got from a proper night sleep because you cannot compensate what you had lost the previous night. It is the sleep and rest the next night that will compensate you and bring freshness to the skin.

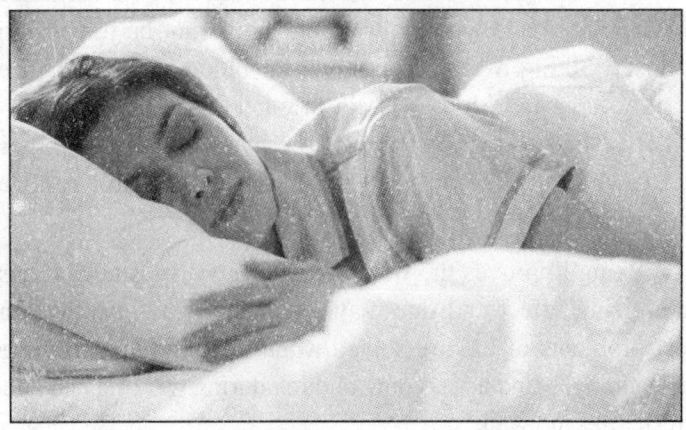

Sleep and rest

I have been touring the whole of India mostly in jeeps, during the whole of my service in Geological Survey of India. I have seen that no driver of the jeep was able to drive more than 100 kilometres at a stretch. He needed rest for a while and whenever I asked them why he needed rest, he would cite the example of the engine of the jeep. "I can drive the vehicle for another 100 kilometers but what about my body-engine? It is getting hot and needs some rest." What a wonderful example of rest!

The engine getting hot would get new life when it cools down. If it were to run continuously, the extent of wear and tear would be more in the engine parts. The same is the case with human machine. It needs not only rest but also sleep to cool down what had become hot during exertions. Our skin is renovated in this fashion.

When a person suffers from some disease and he is on medicines, the first attempt for the doctor is to induce him good sleep. It is only sleep that kills the disease germs, repairs the damaged skin and organs and gives natural strength.

Good Effects of Sleep on the Body

- The skin of the body is nourished and gets new life
- The body temperature decreases. High or immoderate temperature damages the skin
- The heart goes slow
- The blood pressure becomes less
- The rate of respiration becomes less
- The function of the kidneys is regulated and discharges are more. No sleep means no skin health

The skin becomes dry and blood is polluted thus becoming a cause for skin damage.

The digestion is disturbed. Constipation occurs polluting the blood and causing harm to the skin.

How to Improve your Sleep?

- Do not be awake till late night.
- Do not watch television or cinema or read novels till late night.
- Do not allow fear, stress, worry and anger to trouble you when you sleep.
- Do not do excessive exercises; do not over eat and do not observe fast.
- Take your dinner at least 2 hours before you go to bed.
- Take a bath before going to bed (summer).
- Wash your hands and feet before going to bed in winter.
- Take a glass of lukewarm milk before going to bed.
- The bed where you sleep should be comfortable.
- The bedroom should be airy and if there are mosquitoes, a net is essentially to be installed on the bed.
- Do not drink liquor to get the sleep.

According to 'Charak Samhita' (a well-known text on Ayurveda), these are the following measures that induces good sleep:

- Apply and massage the body with oil.
- Apply oil on the head.
- Take a bath with 'Ubtan' (herbal applicant).
- Drink milk, eat yogurt and ghee.
- Only those dishes which one likes in taste should be served.

- A little quantity of alcohol can be taken. Non-vegetarians may take fish and chicken in little quantity.
- Good fragrant flowers should be kept in the bed room and fragrances to be applied on the bed and the body.
- Soft and good music can be played before sleeping.
- A soft bed and an airy atmosphere also helps in achieving good sleep.

Try to avoid keeping your legs towards the east and the south direction while sleeping. You may get disturbed sleep. If these waves enter from the legs, they lighten the work of blood circulation back to heart. This magnetic explanation may not be thought authenticated but there are references of sleep position and direction in the above fashion in the old Vedic books. Sleep in the above direction if you are sleeping otherwise in wrong direction and you will know the difference by yourself. Your sleep will be sound and normal.

(*Note:* Some of the guide-lines given above in 'Charak Samhita' may seem awkward in the present era but it is up to you to decide the feasibility after experimenting with them at the time of sleep)

Sleep and rest are essential parts of life and if one is deprived of this gift of nature, perfect skin will turn into problem skin.

SKIN HEALTH OF BABIES

Baby skin is smooth and soft. It is thin and fragile than an adult's. It is incapable of tolerating extreme hot and cold temperatures. Babies need extra covers in winter. Massaging is very good for babies. It is a traditional therapy for building the body of the baby. It provides good sleep and enhances immunity besides strengthening the muscles. Cleaning the body-folds of a baby

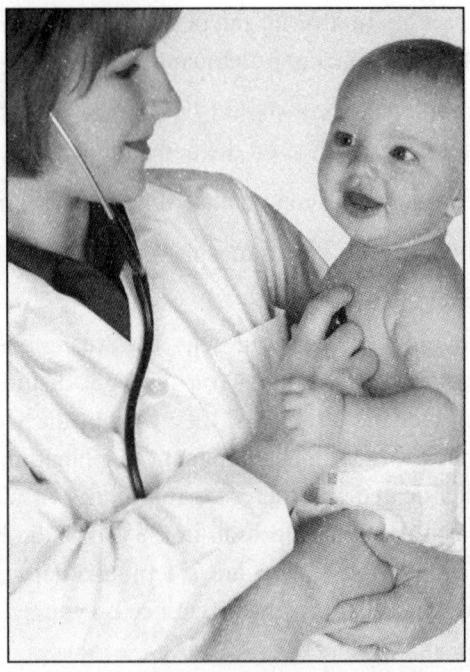

Skin health of babies

is a must. Mothers should clean the folds at the neck, thighs, elbows, beneath the kneecaps, armpits and groins. Infection takes place in these junctions in most of cases. Regular trimming of the fingernails of a baby should be done regularly so he does not damage his own skin by scratching harshly. If you observe some rashes or acne on the face of babies, it maybe due to increased hormonal activity from the mother's blood. Clean the rashes and apply coconut oil. Clean the external ear of the baby every week.

When the baby has slept, put a net over him so that he/she is protected from mosquitoes and flies. Do not apply insect repellent creams or anti-allergic medication on his skin. If round white blisters or bumps appear on the skin due to some insect bite, apply some coconut oil. The markets today are flooded with baby products if one has the time and money to spare. Until and unless there is some problem skin, eruptions, or other complications, the application of coconut oil and the use of a mild soap are the best options. In times of doubt, one should consult a doctor. In this way, the babies will be able to retain their perfect skin and will not face any type of problem skin.

STRESS

Stress is something that is thoroughly interlinked with one another. If someone else is doing something, I maybe getting stressed due to his act. We are faced with some or the other major crisis in life in the form of examinations, interviews, service, unemployment, financial struggles, marriage problems, divorce, family conflicts, bereavement and battling with noise or pollution of big city life. If you are doing something against your will and under pressure of parents or your boss or even friends, you are stressed.

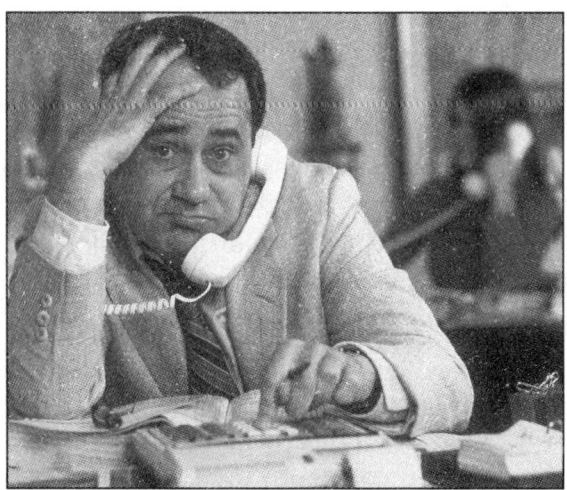

Stress

The boredom of retirement or unemployment also creates stress in the life. The stress of any kind has a direct bearing upon the mental and physical well-being. The physical impact of stress is on skin. Psoriasis is one of the severe skin conditions that have a deep connection with stress and worries. Anxiety, fear, repressed anger and emotions lead to many skin diseases. It may sound strange but it has truth in its depth. Skin diseases have been established due to hereditary disorders, nutritional deficiencies, metabolic disorders, physical induced agents, bacterial infections, and viral infections etc. but it has a serious relation with stress and worry.

If someone is having any one of the above and taking treatment internally or externally but is most confused with his state of the stressed mind, he or she will not recover with any of the methods be it internal or external medicine.

How to Solve Worries and Cure Skin Diseases?

Worries should not be taken to the brains. The worries should be written down in words. Write the problems being faced and then write the possible consequences due to problems. Now write down the solutions as you think best. Be ready to face the eventualities for what you have suggested to yourself and all your worries will be soon evicting your brains. This way the worries are exposed in the real sense. When we think about solutions and consequences of situations arising out of worries, it is a zigzag way. We are already crowded with many other worries and our mind is not having any vacant space to accommodate the recent worry.

Our mind is like a digital calculator where suppose the capacity is for 8 digits then we cannot accommodate the ninth digit in it. For additional workouts, we have to write down ourselves on paper. In the same way, the mind is not exclusively free to solve our 'ninth' worry within itself. We have to write down our worry and the solution comes before us as easily as we had never thought of!

FASTS

Over eating is responsible for most of the diseases that afflict mankind. Tasty meals tempt a man or a woman to eat more than one eats and the human machine has a mechanism in which one knows what to eat and what not to eat.

The idea of observing fast once a week that is one meal a day is helpful for digestion especially when one is aging. The purpose of fasting is to give rest to the stomach. You cannot give rest to your heart but you can give rest to your stomach and the associated digestive organs. By fasting, the internal organs of the abdomen and stomach muscles get rest. Human body is a machinery and it deserves servicing like any other machine. The best way to service this machine is to give it rest. On the day of fast if you opt not to take salt for one day, it is still better. It is a natural fact that the whole week you take salt and salt is also received by the body through many foods. A day's rest for the body to get salt will also help in digestion.

Fasting is a natural method of keeping a person healthy. If you cannot observe even one day fast, limit it to one meal at least. You can take fruits and milk on the day of fasting. In the old age, one should not take heavy meals in the breakfast. Occasionally, heavy food items can be taken but it is better to avoid it. 'Fast' and not going on 'feast' should be the motto of people who are getting old. 'Eat to live' and not 'live to eat' should be the motto to ensure good health.

EXAMINING SKIN HEALTH

We have talked about the conditions of perfect skin which turns into problem skin and then problem skin turning into perfect skin. Here is a study on how the perfect skin can be retained in its perfect condition if some care is taken personally. This care is nothing but involves examining your own body.

As a general trend, we go to the doctors in utmost emergency conditions when the problem of health is beyond one's control of treatment. In this regard, the example of a fire extinguisher can be given. When there is fire in the house and we have a fire extinguisher at hand or water stored for such eventuality, these resources can be used as a precaution. Fire can be extinguished quickly without called for the fire brigade. In the same way, if we have some domestic remedial measures or some medicines handy at home, we can avoid going to doctor.

Even if we do not have such remedial measures at home, we can do something for a proper and timely cure. This is examining your body daily and weekly to find out the abnormalities as detailed below.

DAILY EXAMINATION OF YOUR BODY

Immediately after getting up in the morning, you find yourself yawning frequently. If this is your daily routine, you have to be careful. This might mean that you are not getting good sleep and rest. The skin of the body has not got its nourishment for recouping the luster lost during daytime and harsh climates. Take measures as suggested in the sleep and rest caption in the last chapter. Check your tongue and teeth. If your tongue is white coated and the teeth are yellow, this means there is some digestive problem. Whatever we take in meals, a major part of our digested food converts into sweat, urine, and stool. Some of the undigested contents of the chewed food material travel towards the tongue and oral cavity. It also gets mixed up with the saliva. The teeth and tongue thus get dirty or yellowish. This is mostly due to habit of taking heavy food in dinner, not going for evening or after-dinner walks, sleeping immediately after eating thus giving no time to the digestive system for doing its digestion work.

Poor digestion means changes in the blood circulation and blood has relation with the skin. Your skin is likely to get various affections related to polluted blood. If you find dry marks of saliva on the corners of your mouth or chin after you get up in the morning, it is an indication that there is heavy constipation or worms in the stomach. If you are constipated, take measures as suggested in the last chapter. If there are worms, they change the whole biochemistry of the blood circulation. The blood gets feeble circulation especially in the areas relating to face, neck or chest. As a result there will be white spots appearing on face. In this respect, homeopathy has amazing medicines which can do wonders. Cina 30, can be tried as a first aid. 4 pills three times a day for seven days should be taken. If this does not work, better consult a doctor.

If you find that your outer nose skin area beneath the nose is a little red and rough or irritating, this is indication that you may get cold or fever soon. It maybe that you have undergone different temperatures or taken hot or cold fatty things in excess which the stomach has not been able to digest properly. It is now ready to throw out the debris of food through the passage meant for excretion. Nostrils in the form of watery cold also make discharges. This water makes the nostrils red and the areas near it irritating. (This is excellent theory of Unani and Ayurveda where it is believed that most of colds are due to stomach upset).

If cold (coryza) is the result of cold winds and change of climate, the symptoms will be same as in a stomach upset case. Coryza and cold has a distinct action on skin. The outer nose and the kin beneath the nostrils will have irritation and become rough or reddish. Such a change is continued till the cold lasts. Application of vaseline or some cream lessens the inflammation. Take domestic measures or homoeopathic medicines. I need not explain the domestic measures. These are well-known in our homes. (You can get guidance on all petty disorders and diseases from my book 'Self-healing homoeopathic guide for beginners published by B. Jain Publishers, New Delhi).

If there is coughing in the morning, the reason maybe the climate or digestion. The person who has such a coughing, may have taken lot of food containing excessive fats. The body not being able to digest it tries to throw it out in the form of cough. Contact your doctor immediately and report the complaint. Do not think that it is a minor disorder. If ignored at this stage, it may become a chronic case later. The outcome of cough on the skin is tremendous in some cases. The inguinal hernia in the body is the outcome of harsh and continued coughs. (One of the primary reasons and aggravation of existing hernia).

If there is acne or pimple growth on the face during the age of 13 to 16, we generally blame the hormonal change for this but it is not always so. The constipation and improper digestion is also responsible for acne and boils on the face and back in special.

WEEKLY EXAMINATION OF YOUR BODY

See your face in the mirror minutely and find out if there are any changes in respect to boils, rashes, acne, pimples etc.

Examine your hair. Are they soft and black as they used to be or getting gray? Check the scalp for any dandruff or scaling. Are your hair getting thinner or is there any hair loss or bald spot?

Are you seeing properly with your eyes? Do your eyes look sunken in the sockets? Are there any dark circles around your eyes? Does your vision become temporarily dark, when getting up from your seat? Observe the colour of your eyes; are they red or yellow?

Are you able to hear the way you used to hear last year or a few months back? Are there any discharges from ears? Are there any eruptions on or around ears?

Are all your bone joints working without pains? Do you get some knocking sound from you knees when walking? Are any of the bones of your body protruding on the skin or visibly poking out on the skin?

Do you sometimes stagger while walking? Do you feel heaviness in the upper part of body and you desire to sit down while walking? Do you have burning sensations in the soles? Do you get excessive sweat on your palms and soles? Do you get palpitations and feel suffocated? Do you feel feverish and burning in the eyes? Does your feet and soles become cold at night?

If you are having any one of the above symptoms, consult a doctor immediately before the skin problems carry you further or any other disease comes up. This weekly examination of the body skin is a primary practice to be conducted.

Chapter 6

Cosmetic Care of the Face and the Skin

ARE COSMETICS IMPORTANT?

Cosmetics are considered as a tool to improve and beautify the skin. The market in every city of today's world is flooded with various types of cosmetics for sale which are meant for males and females both. Naturally when these cosmetics are being sold, they possess the safety certificate of the authorities and hence can be called harmless provided, they suit the particular skin of the person. It is up to the customer to check the ingredients of the product whether they are safe or not.

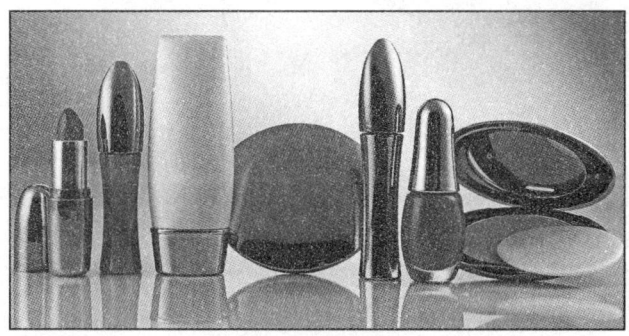

Cosmetics

In the recent times, there has been an increase in the number of beauty parlours and also an increase in the advertising of the cosmetics like soaps, powders, creams, lotions and rouges etc. Millions of people without any care and hesitation are buying these products. How this has happened is also a history. People have become lazy in doing manual work and exercises that can improve their health and in turn the beauty of the face. The natural glow of the face has been robbed due to pollution, wrong type of food-intake, dusty and dirty conditions of working, and of course the disturbed mental condition. To compensate all these wrongs, people are turning towards cosmetics.

MEN CHASE COSMETICS TOO!

It maybe noted that cosmetics are not any more a prerogative of women. Men now chase these equally! The products which are in most demand for men are beauty products like creams, hair gels, lotions, serums, perfumes and anti-aging products. These products of males have higher sales and are considered as the fast moving consumer goods. Their sales have increased tremendously in the recent years. Of all the products, the sale of men's fairness cream has gone very high due to the rigorous advertisement campaigns on television and the print media. Next to the fairness creams

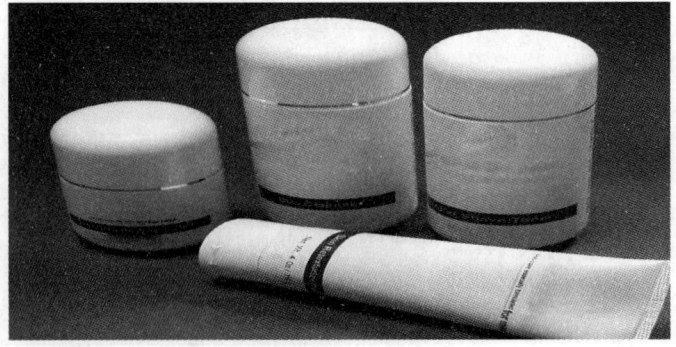

Men's cosmetics

are anti-aging solutions that are selling fast. The third segment that has recently come up are the products that take care of the nails and hands. Manicured hands and well-groomed looks are fascinating men now. Naturally, when film personalities are advocating the fairness creams, men are likely to be attracted to the domain of women. Good looks mean shaving creams, razors, anti-dandruff shampoos, talcum powders, toothpastes and deodorants.

WHICH COSMETICS ARE THE MOST USED?

Cosmetics are made of two major constituents, chemicals and herbs (including kitchen additives). Some of the products have pure chemicals, some contain pure herbs, and most of them are mixture of chemicals and herbs. Let us take creams first that are used by both males and females. These creams serve more purpose of shine and wax than actual moistening or drying the skin according to the quality of cream. Next comes the cleanser. They can also be called creams that clean the face and the body. Within the cleansers category come soap, and scrubs. Cosmetic care of face does not mean care of skin or face with the help of beauty products that are generally called cosmetics.

Cosmetic is a substance for beatifying the complexion and improving the appearance. There are many cosmetics available in the market and people mostly depend upon them after seeing advertisements in the magazines, newspapers, and television. We shall not discuss about the cosmetics available in the market but cosmetics in the real sense that can be prepared at home. On the other hand, we have alternative treatment other than allopathy. Homoeopathic suggestions and Ayurvedic preparations are quite efficient tools to improve upon the skin and complexion.

SIDE EFFECTS OF COSMETICS NOT SUITING THE SKIN

There are many persons who purchase cosmetics but find them allergic to their skin. In such cases, people have to change the particular brand of cream or lipstick etc. and go to the doctor for the rashes or allergy spots. Homoeopathy has very good medicines to cure such cases where cosmetics have reacted with the skin adversely.

People have a tendency to purchase advertised cosmetics for acne and other skin problems and incidentally if they do not suit the skin, they generally harm the skin and the condition of acne or other problems becomes worse. In such cases, the use of that particular cosmetic/cream, lotion etc. should be stopped. Taking Bovista 30, a homoeopathic medicine, 4 pills three times a day for seven days removes the ill effects of cosmetics.

HERBAL COSMETICS

The present era is full of cosmetics for enhancing the beauty of the face. The top on the Indian list is herbal cosmetics. Indians faithfully follow the herbal phenomenon. Away from laser treatments or cosmetic surgeries, our belief is more in herbal treatments and perhaps that is why this book has a number of formulae in herbal treatments for various skin problems. The most striking fact is that this Indian herbal faith is not limited in the Indian continent but has spread more in Europe and USA too. There were a number of herbal creams who bombarded the television screen with their advertisements until the coming of the well-known 'Shehnaz Hussain' who rocked the country and also won accolades in the international markets with her beauty products. This was the onset of fame related to herbal products in India.

In every beauty parlour, you will find products like 24-carat gold, pearl, astro gems therapy and diamond collection. Not only the upper classes were fascinated with these herbal creams and lotions but the middle class also gets their brands at cheaper rates. Besides 'Shehnaz', we have Vandana Luthra's 'Curves and Curls' (VLCC), Lotus herbal, Biotech, Himalayas, Ayur, Cadilla, Beiersdorf, Hamburg (Nivea products), and Nicholas Piramal etc. in the market on competitive prices.

Before proceeding to the care and treatment of face, it is essential that we know the texture of our facial skin. There are many women who are ignorant about the texture of their skin and purchase various skin creams from the market or conduct homemade solutions or creams that do not give favourable results to their skin. I have observed that many girls or women coming to my clinic do not know to which category of skin they have. Those girls who are aware of the texture of their skin are educated and hence read about the skin care. For women who do not actually know the texture of their skin, it becomes difficult for me to prescribe the medicine. A test of self-observation is then given to the patient and when it is over, she knows the texture. I am describing this test for the benefit of the readers.

We have generally three types of skin textures and this is obviously related to the face. These types are oily, dry and mixed (oily/dry). At first we will have a self-observation test and then a practical test.

OILY SKIN TEST

Observe the following on your face:

- The face of an oily-skinned person has a shining appearance.
- Its pores are widely open and the blackheads and whiteheads are visible.

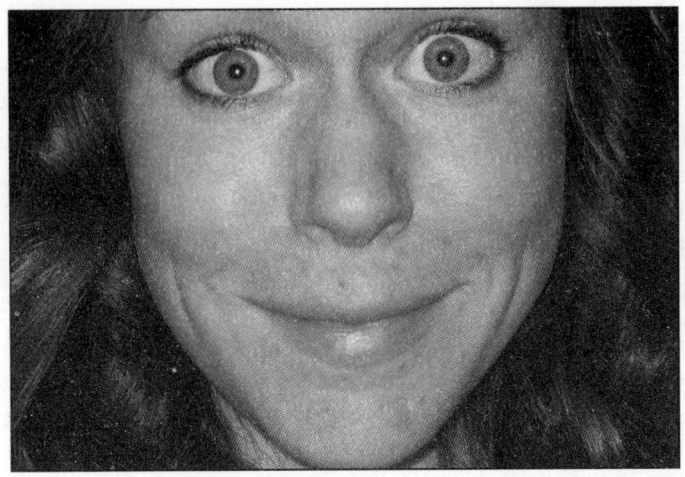

Oily skin

- The texture of oily skin is coarse, thick and slightly yellow.
- Oily skin attracts more of dirt and so external influences do react with them.
- Acne, pimples and boils are common for them. It is due to over activity of the sebaceous glands that produce excessive oil secretions.
- It has relation with hormonal activity of the body as well.

DRY SKIN TEST

Observe the following on your face:

- Dry skin is sensitive with flaky patches. Its pores are not visible.
- Dry skin is more prone to develop wrinkles. If not treated adequately, it gives a look of premature old skin.
- Dry skin may have thyroid problems.

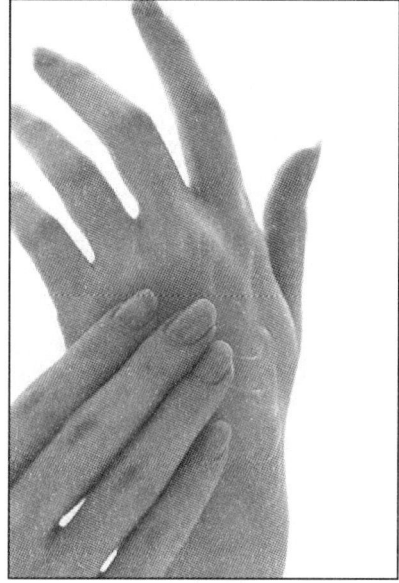

Dry skin

- In summer, dry skin people may have chaps on the face.
- Such a texture brings premature lines in the corner of eyes and mouth.
- Persons with dry skin are less prone to those skin diseases relating to sweat glands.
- Dry skin people tend to get eczema and allergic rashes
- Even the slight scratch with the nails on the skin can bring in red streaks on the dry-skin persons. This streak disappears after a short time.
- Dry skin condition is due to under activity or sluggish activity of oil glands. The secretion of oil from the skin is insufficient to grease the skin.
- Excessive use of soaps, cosmetics and lack of nutritional food

and over exposure to the sun are the major reasons for dry skin.

MIXED OILY AND DRY SKIN TEST

The third structural category of skin texture is not oily or dry facial skin but a mixture of both. Observe the following on your face:

- This mixed facial skin has partly oily and partly dry.
- In most of the cases the forehead, nose and the chin in a straight line (vertically) look oily but the other parts of the face appears dry.
- Partly oily and partly dry skin is due to the malfunctioning of the sweat glands. There is less of water and the condition of dehydration is there in the body.

HEALTHY SKIN OF THE FACE

We have learnt about three types of skins, dry, oily and mixed. There are people who have healthy skin on the face. The test is very simple. Persons who do not feel any kind of stretched sensation on

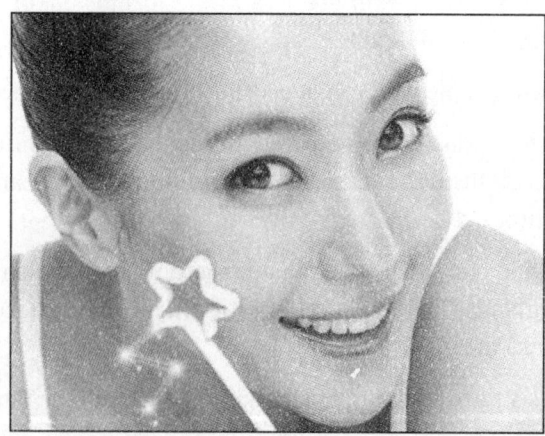

Healthy skin of the face

their face and the face is free of any skin disorder are those blessed with a naturally healthy and beautiful skin.

Practical test

Checking texture of your skin

Now that you have observed your face with the above tests and found you have a dry skin, oily skin, or mixed skin.

Here is the practical test now:

- Get some tissue paper. Fold it in strips.
- Early in the morning without washing your face, rub and slide the strips to and fro gently over your nose, forehead, chin and cheeks.
- Now check the strips. If there are some stains of grease, your skin is oily.
- If there are no stains and the strips remain unchanged, your skin is dry.
- Next morning, without washing the face, rub and slide a strip on the centre of your face starting from you forehead to nose and chin. Then see the strip carefully.
- Now take another strip and rub/slide it on cheeks and surrounding areas. Check the strip.
- In the above two tests, if the strips differ from each other, that means the central part of your face is oily and the sides are dry. You have a mixed skin.

Care of oily faces

It is a known fact that oily skin is difficult to handle because it attracts most of the dust and polluted substances from the air. A strict routine of cleaning the oily face has to be maintained. The face and the neck should be washed a number of times during a day and especially when one returns from outdoor activities like shopping or an outing. The makeup applied during the daytime has to be removed meticulously when one returns from outside and it has to be wiped off completely while going to bed.

During summers, do not use creamy or fat-enriched creams or beauty soaps. The soap should be mild and medicated. The soap should produce a lot of lather which should be rinsed with fresh water. Clean your face with cotton wool dipped in good quality cleansing lotion. Alternatively, some freshener (the type we get in air travels) can also be used. Those who are having pitting on the face or have old scars as a result of acne rosacea should use an astringent to tone and tighten the pores. Using rose water on the face at night is very beneficial for people with oily skin.

Care of dry faces

Dry skin of a face does not need meticulous regime for caring until it is affected with a skin disease. At night, the people with dry skin may use creams with fats and oil. The soaps having glycerin and useful fats should be used for cleaning the face. After returning from outside, dry skin people should also wash their face with a good oily soap and then dry it with cotton soaked with a freshener. A good oil based cream then can be applied spreading all over the face lavishly.

Treatment of oily skin

- Excess intake of nutritional supplements associated with some food allergy leads to oily skin.
- If additional supplements have been taken, the skin blemishes may appear on the face.
- Excessive Iodine may also produce oily skin and triggers acne, pimples. Such persons having oily skin with acne or pimples should avoid use of iodine-salt.

Cosmetic Care of the Face and the Skin

- The foremost care and treatment for oily skin people is to maintain cleanliness.
- A person with oily skin should wash his/her face three to four times daily.
- It is always beneficial to wash the face, apply a little lemon juice, keep it for two minutes and washing it off with fresh water.
- Taking hot steam on the face at least thrice weekly is essential to remove blackheads. Intake of 10,000 units of Vitamin A (consult doctor for the quantity) is said to be useful for people having oily skin. But the consumption of vitamin A in the form of vegetables or fruits is definitely a better option.

Homoeopathy offers wonderful medicines for oily, greasy and shining skin. They are Nat-m, Plb., Psor., Sanic., and Thuja. The medicines should be taken under the guidance of doctor.

Treatment of dry skin

- Get your 'Thyroid profile' tested by a laboratory after consulting a doctor. Thyroid trouble is one of the main reasons for dry skin.
- In many people, dry skin leads to eczema of the body and it is generally accompanied by some food allergy that initiates or increases the existing eczema. A doctor should be consulted.
- Daily oil massage of the whole of body should be done in winter. Less the use of soap in winter, the better it is for the skin.
- In winter people with dry skin may use heated vaporizers in their bedroom at night to maintain high level of humidity.
- Diet should have adequate fats.

MASSAGE OF THE FACE

Today the markets are flooded with innumerable cosmetic massage creams, face creams, lotions and soaps in the market to help us do our cosmetic care. They are supposed to help preserve the beauty and youthfulness of the skin. But sadly enough, all are not beneficial to everyone.

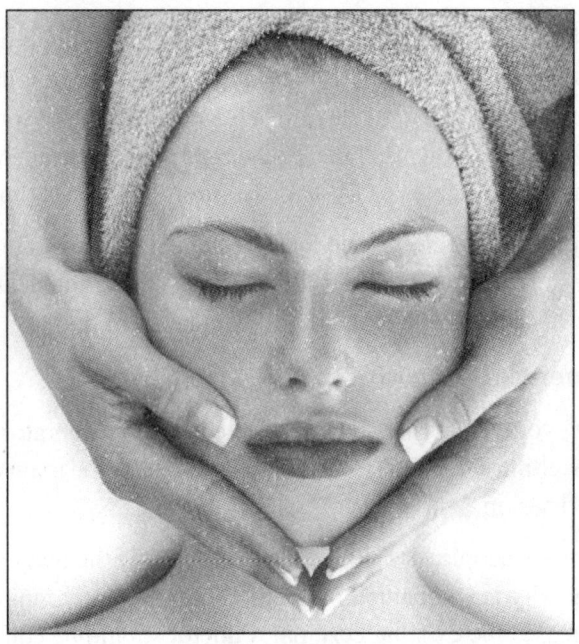

Massage of the face

Everyone has a different skin pattern and hence all the creams or aids are not useful for all skin types. Along with massaging of the face there are two more ways of enhancing the beauty of facial skin and that is *cupping* and *steaming*. Facial massage is meant to tone up a relaxed skin, improve the texture and fade away the wrinkles. There is a popular belief that that massage removes deposits of fat on the face especially of those who have double chin. Massaging with appropriate type of creams, followed by soap and water is believed to maintain the attractiveness of a face.

Along with massage, there is need for cleaning the skin and warming the skin; and for this cupping and steaming is done. These assist in the stimulation and improvement of the circulation of blood in the skin. Those who have greasy skin or skin with blackheads, the massage is useful. But if the same skin conditions also have boils, acne with pus formation, the infection may spread by massaging. In such cases, massaging should be avoided.

Types of Face Massage

The latest in the beauty parlours is the plastic massage of Jacquet (a trade mark), which is a violent form of massage and must be given by a physician.

General Massage of the Face at Night

The most common known massage of the face is done at night by most of the ladies before retiring to bed. In this type, one applies the required quantity of a suitable cream with the help of right hand thumb and two fingers. A light pressure is made on the face while rubbing and gliding. In rubbing and gliding one should follow the normal folds of the skin. A massage of five to ten minutes is sufficient for this type of massaging. If you have no knowledge of such a course of rubbing, you can observe the same when you get your facial done from a beauty parlour. It is easy to learn from the way, the expert's make the to and fro or up-down strokes on your face.

When you get the facial done at a beauty parlour, see that the person doing your facial has washed his or her hands and cleaned the apparatus.

FACIAL MASSAGE AT HOME

If you are unable to learn/imitate from the technique used at the beauty parlour, here is some of the procedure to guide you:

First Method

- Smear your hands and face with plenty of good face cream.
- Start a light massage from the frontal neck, upwards to the chin and jaw bones with the help of fingers of both your hands. Do these strokes lightly for at least eight to ten times.
- With the help of back of your hands, slap the muscles of your chin for ten times. This is a good action for reducing fat of double chin.
- Massage your cheeks by making strokes with your hands towards temples and backstroke towards cheeks. Now massage your eyes over the eyelids and then give a light massage under the eyes moving your hands from outer corners of the eyes towards the inner corners.
- The third step is to move your fingers around the eyes in the clockwise direction and then in the anticlockwise direction.
- Give a good massage to your nose moving your fingers in a circular fashion. Start massaging from the bridge of the nose to tip.

Second Method

- Smear your hands with plenty of a good face cream.
- With the fingers of your both hands make a circular motion on the face from chin towards side of the eye passing through the cheeks, forehead and the side of the other eye, other cheek and back to the chin. Massage with a gentle touch both in the clockwise and anticlockwise direction five times each.

- With the help of the middle finger and the ring finger of both the hands, start massaging from the corner of the left side of the lips to the left side of the nose to right side of the eyebrow. Cover the eyebrow and return from left side of eyebrow back to the lips corner. The same rotational massage is to be done from the right side of lips at the same time. Do it for five times.

- With the fingers of both the hands massage beneath both the eyes in a to and fro fashion for ten times.

- With the middle and the ring fingers of both the hands, massage on the corner of both eyes in a circular way for five times.

- Now massage around the eyes in a circular fashion ten times, in a clockwise and anticlockwise fashion.

- Spread your right hand index and middle finger in the shape of 'V' and place the fingers on the right side of the forehead. Now place the index finger of the left hand in the middle of the two fingers of the right hand and massage the forehead to and fro for ten times.

- Tap all the fingers of both your hands on the forehead as is done while playing the 'tabla' (a musical instrument).

- With the fingers of both the hands, make to and fro massage motion from the nose towards the head for ten times and from head towards nose for ten times.

- Keep the index and the middle finger of the left hand on the chin and pull the skin downwards. Now with the help of the index and the middle finger of right hand, massage the cheek in a circular fashion, both clockwise and anti-clockwise ten times each. Repeat the same on the other cheek.

- Put both your hands on the neck and massage the neck upwards.

- After the massage is done, wipe your face with the help of wet cotton pieces and then apply some face pack.

Steaming the Face

The procedure of steaming involves evaporation of steam on the face to cleanse the pores of the skin and increase the sweat. Steaming activates the sweat glands. This should be done by professionals but if you are acquainted with it and learnt it, it can be done at home on weekly basis.

Boil some water in a vessel and put the bowl beneath your face. Cover the face and head with a towel so that the steam coming out of the utensil does not escape. Close your eyes and let the steam touch you're the whole of your face. As and when you feel very hot, suffocating, remove the towel from head, and suspend the steaming for a while. Wipe your face with clean towel and repeat the steaming for a while again. After you have taken the steam twice, apply cold cream or some powder on the face.

Cupping the Face

Cupping of face is a procedure that is done in the beauty clinic with the help of apparatus. Cupping is also used as a term for normalising the colour of the dark circles around the eyes. In this method of cupping, the palms of both the hands are rubbed against each other vigourously and when they become hot, the palms are kept on the eyes making a cup with the hands. The heat generated by rubbing is thus released all over and around the eyes making a smoothening effect both on the skin and the vision of the eyes. This activity also stimulates the circulation of blood in the skin especially the around eyes and helps remove dark circles if done regularly at night.

The term cupping is referred to with a different term in the beauty parlours. Technically, it is a term used by cosmetic experts.

This is a procedure to mildly suck the skin. The cups meant for the function of sucking are boiled and its rims are cleaned thoroughly with alcohol with during the time of application. A rubber bulb is attached to the cup which produces the suction. The cup is smeared from within (inner surface) with alcohol and put on the face. The suction is started and the skin is sucked mildly so as not to cause pain. The suction should take place for two to four minutes. The cupping is stated to cleanse the pores of the skin, activate the sweat glands and extract foreign particles from the skin, if there are any. Many skin experts think that steaming is better than cupping.

COSMETIC CARE PREPARATIONS AT HOME FOR OILY SKIN

Fuller's Earth as Cleaning Scrubs

Fullers' earth is a mineral useful for the skin. Fuller's earth is also one variety of fuller's earth. Since ages, this has been in used by women to enhance their beauty.

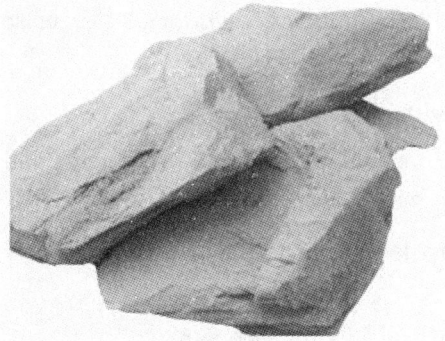

Fuller's earth

The Best Cleaning Scrub for Face

- First of all take one-fourth cup of orange peel. Dry it and grind it into powder.

- Mix it with one-fourth cup of fuller's earth and two teaspoonful of sandalwood powder. This can be stored in a jar for your use.
- While taking a bath, take one teaspoonful of this mixture and make a paste by adding some water. Apply this paste on your face and wait for five minutes. Now rinse it with a little warm water.
- This mixture of fuller's earth can remove pimples and acne. But for this you have to mix half teaspoon of margosa powder (leaves of a mahogany variety) to the paste before applying on the face. Rest of the procedure is same.
- The above mixtures should be used at least every alternate day to get the desired effect.

Cleansing Mask with Fuller's Earth

- Take one-fourth cup of fuller's earth and add some tomato pulp
- Keep this mixture aside
- Take two tablespoonful of yogurt and one teaspoonful of cucumber juice
- Mix them thoroughly
- Mix both the first and second mixtures together and mix them thoroughly to make a paste; the mask is ready
- Apply this mask on your face and wait for fifteen to twenty minutes.
- Rinse the mask away with cold water
- Every third day this mask should be applied for a beautiful shining face

TONERS

Vinegar for a Glowing Face

- If your face is of dry type, prepare a mixture with half teaspoonful of vinegar and half teaspoonful of lemon juice.
- Put some drops of rose water in this mixture and apply on your face.
- Wash the face with little warm water when your face feels dry; you will find your face glowing.

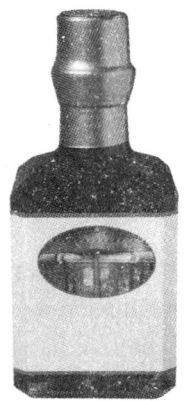
Vinegar

Body Toners

- Body toners are to bring a glow to the skin and keep the skin colour normal and harmonised. Toners are available in the market also but here is a toner that is very handy for the use at home. These toners can be used frequently during the daytime at home.
- Mix one teaspoonful of cabbage juice with an equal quantity of rose water.
- Add a pinch of alum in it. It can be stored if made proportionately.
- The same mixture can be made by substituting cabbage juice with cucumber juice.

Non-vegetarian Toner Mask for the Face

- Take one tablespoon of yogurt and one tablespoon of fuller's earth. Mix them.
- Take one egg and extract the white of it.
- Add this white of egg and mix thoroughly with yogurt and fuller's earth.

- Apply this on your face and let it dry.
- After it is dry, rinse it off with clean water. Do not let it remain on your face after the mixture gets dry.
- The mask can be applied every fourth day.

HOME-MADE PREPARATIONS FOR DRY SKIN

The primary action and care for dry skin is to keep it nourished and moisturised regularly. Persons with dry skin should not go much in the sun, harsh winds and hot water baths. They should not use toners that contain alcohol or astringent. They should use soaps that have a lot of fat. Oil based creams should be used. In the market many cold creams and moisturizers are available but here are some hints for making them at home.

Milk Cleanser

Cleansing milk is generally used to clean the face and the pores of skin. Before any cream is applied, it is better to apply cleansing milk so that the pores of skin are free of dirt.

- Take half a cup of milk and warm it a little.
- Add one teaspoonful of glycerin. Mix it well.
- To this mixture, now add one-fourth teaspoon each of bicarbonate soda and borax.
- Dissolve them thoroughly and add some rose water for fragrance. Store in a bottle in cool place.
- Apply this cleansing milk on the face and clean the face with the help of cotton buds. The face will look fresh and the skin will glow.

Cleansing Mask

The purpose of a cleansing mask is to clean the pores of the skin.

- Take a banana and mash it well.
- Take a teaspoon of ghee (a thick fatty substance made from milk cream) and mix into the mashed banana. Mix it completely.
- Apply this paste on the face and let it dry for 15-20 minutes.
- Rinse the mask with the help of cold water. Using it once a week is sufficient.

Moisturizer

As the name indicates, the purpose of a moisturizer is to keep the skin moisturized. A moisturizer available in the market has Aqua paraffinum, liquidium, Alcohol denot, Stearic acid, Myristyi, Coco-glycerides and many other chemicals. Every company has different herbal/chemical ingredients.

Among moisturizers, many use another product called 'Lacto calamine'. It has glycerin and light kaolin (a sort of clay). It is supposed to retain the natural moisture of the skin, protect the face from pollution and removes the dead cells.

- Take one teaspoon of vinegar and mix it with well with one-fourth teaspoon of honey.
- Take half cup of glycerin and an equal quantity of rose water. Mix them both. Then mix vinegar and honey mixture in the same.
- Store it in a bottle and use it after milk cleansers or a cleansing mask.

Chapter 7

Care of Complexion

In the olden days, women used to take help of herbs to beautify their skin and complexion. The perfumes we use today had a different look. In India, they used to apply various abstracts of flowers and oils. The bathing used to be with 'shikakai' (an ayurvedic medicinal plant) and flower essences. They used the oil of sandal and coconut for their complexion and hair. The lipstick was not there but a special type of tree bark (musag) was used to colour the lips. This tree is still available in Jammu and Kashmir (a state in India). Women there still use this bark. To give a pink glow to their cheeks, the women of the olden era in India used sandalwood powder mixed with rose oil.

In the Moghul era, Moghul queens were very fond of using these indigenous cosmetics for the upkeep of their complexion. Fruits were also used in those days for beautification. Fruits were consumed in plenty and also used as face packs. The present day women who live in the countryside still use those time-tested prescriptions. To decrease the swelling around the eyes, raw potatoes cut in circular shapes and placed on the eyes gives relief. Pieces of cucumber and muskmelon are also used for the same purpose.

These days people use makeup armaments like blush on, eye shadow, liner, mascara, lipstick, etc. at home or go to beauty parlors to enhance their beautify. But the best way is the natural way with the help of domestic ingredients.

Life is full of colours. In nature, we have colourful flowers, green vegetation, blue sky, blue sea, white clouds and so on. In this world, people are often identified by their colour. Complexion is of the colour of the skin often assessed by its clarity and its tone.

The skin has a texture. Texture is how you feel the skin when you touch it. Colour is actually deep in the protoplasmic areas of the epidermis. The external epidermal layers are made of transparent flat epithelial cells that shrivel up into polymorphous scales as they approach the surface which are constantly thrown off and are constantly renewed from below. This change is almost invisible.

The skin colour or complexion actually comes from a natural pigment called melanin. The pigment of the skin is a complex chemical substance, the exact constitution of which is not known. It is produced in the cells of the basal layer of the epidermis by the action of an oxidizing ferment on a colourless substance allied to tyrosin and adrenalin. It is actually in the form of fine brownish granules that tend to become aggregated.

Complexion is influenced by age, sex, race, health and climate.

Pollution and extreme weather conditions cause harm to the complexion, causing cell damage, dehydration and pigmentation. Genes and age are two prominent factors which influences the complexion. These two factors of age and genes cannot be changed or altered. Genetic factor is permanent, immutable and changeless. Different races of people have different gene codes, different number of oil and sweat glands, different colour of eyes, hair and skin. These things often help us to identify a particular race. We can easily identify an Asian, European, Chinese and Africans by their features and complexion. The age as we know is an irreversible process of the body.

In the middle and the old age, skin texture becomes dry, thin, and loose. The normal cell renewal during the young age becomes slower and this process gets even more retarded as the old age advances. But this is not all. We have other factors for the damage of complexion and for that we are responsible ourselves. We face it due to our wrong upkeep of the body. Two factors in this process are mostly harmful and they are dry and oily skins.

DARK COMPLEXION AND BEAUTY

Complexion is a gift of God. It maybe fair or dark. Actually, a person maybe beautiful with any type of complexion—fair or dark. Dark complexion is more attractive than the fair one if the features of the face are sharp and in the correct proportion. Dark complexion has its own advantages. On this complexion, wrinkles on the face develop slowly than fair complexioned faces. The sunburns on this face are less visible. The aging of the face comes at a slower pace than fair- complexioned people. Dark complexion has more of strong facial muscles. The irony is that every dark girl or a boy desires to become fair.

Given below is a tip that can improve your complexion. Try it.

Mix one teaspoon of limejuice with an equal quantity of hydrogen peroxide and apply the same on your face. Let it dry and then wash the face. Do it daily before taking a bath for months together and see the difference.

Note: If oily skin is not properly cleaned, it may change

the colour of the skin and even result in blemishes or acne and pimples.

If dry skin is not properly cared for its nourishing or moisturizing are not done at the right time, there maybe eruptions like eczema, scales, and the complexion might become dusky, dirty and dull.

SELECTION OF WRONG BEAUTY PRODUCTS

The markets today are flooded with creams and lotions that claim the lightening or brightening the overall complexion along with lightening the age spots, liver spots, freckles, sun damage, tans, acne marks, old scars and skin discoloration and even birthmarks. But are they effective? This is the question that should be asked. They have a tremendous psychological impact since you have spent money on these products and partly because they work but not to the extent you expect them to work. A lot of dedication, time and patience are needed because your particular skin may not suit the components of the cream or lotion from which the product is actually made. So it is very essential that you select the proper products to ensure that the product you are buying befits your skin type.

If the skin is oily and the product purchased has oil rich contents, it will further add to the woes of the skin. If the skin is dry and the product purchased has medicated contents and a strong astringent to make the skin further dry, the skin may get further damaged.

There are some creams in the market that claim to have the ability of converting black complexion into white. One should be aware and note the chemicals that the product is made of. If the fairness cream is having a mercury drug preparation, the cream may cause discoloration of the skin in patches while going in the sun.

IMPACT OF ANAEMIC CONDITION ON COMPLEXION

If the person is anaemic and has an impaired blood circulation, he or she is likely to have a yellowish-dull complexion. Yellow complexion is also due to jaundice but we know that after jaundice is over, the normal complexion returns. But there are people who are anaemic and do not know it. They have dull pale complexion and go on blaming cosmetics for it. Anaemia also develops dark circles under the eyes. Instead of trying various cosmetics, anaemic people should consult a doctor for their anaemia.

IMPACT OF ACNE AND PIMPLES ON COMPLEXION

If a severe onset of acne and pimples are left on the face for a long period, they could leave scars and pits on the skin. Naturally, this would amount to the change of texture and colour of the facial skin. It is hence essential that acne and pimples be treated in time. We have a separate topic on acne in the next chapter and shall discuss about it there elaborately.

IMPACT OF POOR BLOOD CIRCULATION AND HORMONAL DISTURBANCE

Girls and women having poor blood circulation and irregular menstrual periods are likely to have blemishes, dark circles around eyes and freckles. If the above conditions prevail for a long time, such persons people should consult the doctor.

IMPACT OF FOOD ON COMPLEXION

Diet has a great part to play where your skin and complexion is concerned. If you opt to eat late at night or eat frequently in between meals, there maybe some effect on the complexion due to irregular diet habit. If you indulge in excessive intake of sweets, fried and starchy foods, it may make the skin oily.

SUN SHINE OR SUNBURNS AND COMPLEXION

SPF Factor and Sunscreen Creams

Summers in the countries where the heat, warmth and sunshine increases beyond measure have their markets flooded with sun protection creams. Every good cream has a logo of sun protection factor (SPF) written on it. SPF is a measuring unit to combat sunshine. SPF is a useful armament to judge the capacity to fight against sunshine in USA and Europe but not in India. The skin of the Indians have enough pigments to combat the harmful effects of the ultraviolet rays of the sun. It is also susceptible to tanning that cannot be prevented but the skin never gets burnt. This is the reason that Indians having skin cancer is very rare.

There have been studies on this aspect recently and it is found there is little connection of getting skin cancer due to excessive sunshine or due to deficiency of vitamin D in the body. (Courtesy Reader's Digest-April 2008- vitamin Myth) According to a report published in 'Mail Today' newspaper (April 1, 2008). SPF of 15 is enough if you want to protect your skin from the sun, unless you have some skin disease. A sunscreen that has higher SPF than 15 is marginally more effective. The formula says that higher the SPF, more the chemicals present in the sunscreen. People having a sensitive skin, a sunscreen with higher than 15 SPF can do more harm than good and this may cause acne, rashes and allergy on the skin.

Sunshine is important for the skin and that too skin that is oily and full of acne. Excessive sun tanning causes wrinkles of the skin. India is a hot country and sun tanning is not practiced frequently. In winter and in the mountains where sun disappears for a number of days, sunshine is always welcomed.

In Europe if sun tanning is carried out for a great length of time, it even leads to skin cancer for those who are susceptible to it. One function of sunshine is its capability to provide vitamin D needs of the body. Vitamin D regulates the use of calcium, magnesium, and phosphorus in our bodies. Due to lack of vitamin D, one maybe affected with rickets, retarded growth, and tooth decay in childhood causing osteoporosis (brittle bones) in the old age.

In the middle age, it helps physical well-being and emotional health besides reversal of osteoporosis. Talking about sunburns, there is a myth that sunburn may fade into a tan. It maybe noted that sunburn is a burn and not a pre-requisite state for skin-tan. The sunburn would be ending in damaging the skin. There would be redness and eventually the skin may peel too. Any amount of sun exposure makes an impact on the skin and as we have studied above, it may also result in skin cancer. Premature aging may also be due to excessive exposure to sunlight and sunburns. There is a myth that dark skinned people do not need sunlight protection/screen. Let us be clear that lighter skins have less melanin. Melanin as we have studied above is capable of absorbing UV radiation and protects skin. People with light skin are more sensitive to the effects of UV rays from the sun but people with dark skins have an equal risk or may have more risk by UV radiation. The American Academy of Dermatology recommends routine sunscreen use for dark skinned people. Let us have a look on how to save the skin from sunburns and heat during summer.

Save Your Skin from Sunburns

When you are required to go out in the sun, drink plenty of water. Better carry a water bottle with you.

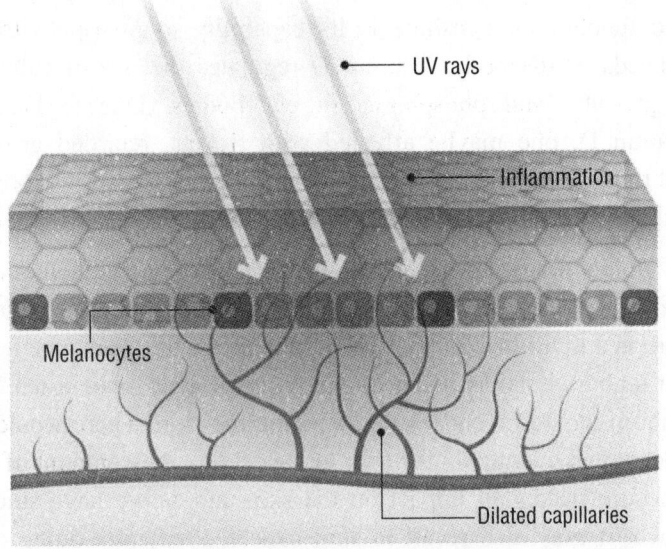

Save your skin from sunburns

- Keep lip-gloss stick, hand sanitizer, a mouth freshener, wet-wipes or facial tissue papers, and small perfume bottle and suitable goggles in your bag while going out in the sun (for ladies only).
- If you want to use a sunscreen cream, apply it at least half an hour before you step out into the sun because it takes that long for the chemicals to penetrate through the skin. After two hours, the sunscreen becomes useless even it is of higher SPF.
- For oily skin, it is better to use gel-based sunscreen.
- If you have tendency to sweating profusely, you are likely

to loose a lot of potassium and sodium. You should have a drink of electrolyte solution when you reach back your home. Electrolyte packs are available with the chemists.

- Wear light coloured clothes or better wear white clothes because it has the capacity to reflect the light back. Clothes of cotton or polyester blends maybe preferred because they can breathe.

- Do not go in the sun all of a sudden when you have been sitting in the air-conditioned room. Similarly do not enter directly or immediately from sun light in the air-conditioned room. Take some time out when in the sun and sometime in when in the room so that your body is acclimatized slowly to the environment you are leaving and entering.

- Take an umbrella or wear a hat to protect from the sun heat. Wear a pair of goggles. The hat should be such that it gives shade to the neck also. If the sunburns have formed on the skin, apply a mixture of yogurt, sandalwood powder and fuller's earth for some days before going to take bath and after the mixture applied is dry, take a bath.

Home-made Sunscreen Lotion

Take one-teaspoon of juice of cucumber, add half teaspoon of glycerin and quantity few drops of rose water. Mix them and keep in the refrigerator to cool. Whenever you go out in the sun, apply this lotion on your face to protect yourself from sunlight.

Water-intake

There is a general concept that people who drink more water generally have a good complexion. Drinking large amount of water without being thirsty is not desired. One should drink more water but not large amounts of water just for the sake of the theory that water is good for health. I have seen people drinking only four or five glasses of water in winter and seven to eight glasses of water in summer and doing quite well with their health. In case of diseases like diabetes or other ailments, if one wants to consume large quantity of water, he or she should consult a doctor for his intake.

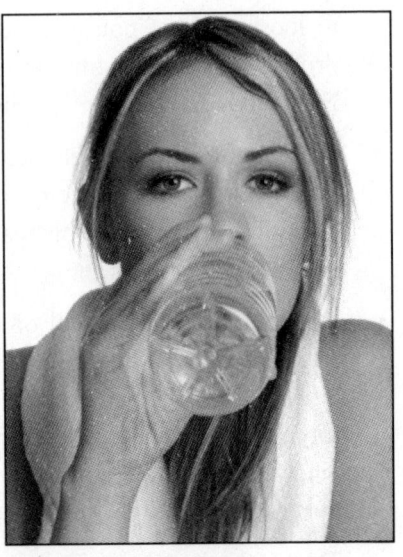

Drink water only when thirsty

Similarly, if there is digestive disturbance, say, acidity, the intake of water will vary. In such a case, a doctor has to be consulted. As food and air are essential for survival, so is water. Our body has 60 percent of water in it. The drinking capacity of water varies according to the climate and constitution of a body.

On an average, our body consumes about 3 to 4 kg of water in 24 hours. This water may not be in the form of water but maybe in the form of food, juices and vegetables. About 30 percent of water reaches our stomach in the form of food. Our body produces about 9 percent of water, and the rest of the water is consumed. Whatever water goes inside, the same quantity is drained out of body in the form of urine, stool, spit, skin and breath.

According to the legend, good intake of water is supposed to make the complexion smooth and fair but recent scientific research has nothing to prove this. The body has 60 percent water and the extra intake of water will not make much impact on the complexion. According to a report published in the Journal of the

American Society of Nephrology, excessive water intake ensures more trips to the toilet. This maybe a study in accordance with nephrology. However, the impact of water on the complexion is a controversial subject.

ALCOHOL

Alcohol is the most harmful, hateful and heartless drink. It has a complex nature of effects on the skin besides its bad effect on over all health. Those who drink regularly, their skin is more prone to develop folds and wrinkles. There will be an artificial reddish colour on the skin due to liquor intake but the inner health of the skin will be deteriorating day by day. This reddish colour will turn blackish and yellowish once the liver is affected with alcohol.

SMOKING

Tobacco has a substance called 'Nicotine'. It is reasonably poisonous and harmful for health. If tobacco in a concentrated form is dissolved in water and given to horse or dog for drinking, it can kill them. In the human body, it dissolves with the blood and creates many chronic diseases of skin, asthma, tuberculosis, and even cancer. Cigarette smokers have skin problems on their fingers and lips. The fingers and lips of the smokers develop yellow patches, which do not go even after leaving smoking. These yellow stains are almost permanent.

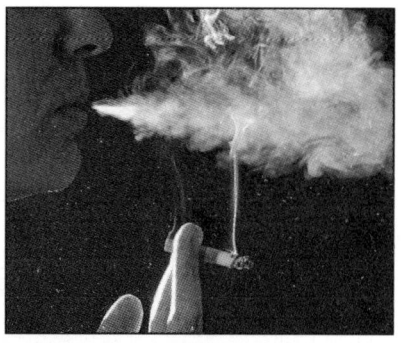
Smoking

If you lack will power to discard smoking you may consult a

Homoeopath. Homoeopathy works on the symptoms of an individual. It is no more a faith healing system but a scientific doctrine based on definite principles. Its tiny sugar pills do not help in fighting a disease but help build vital force in the body. There is no specific remedy to eradicate an addiction but Daphne Indica, Tabacum, Opium, Caladium, and Plantago are some of the medicines, which are helpful.

TEA OR COFFEE

There was time when tea or coffee was not known in the Indian villages. The world of publicity has done a lot for these two items. Now there is not a single house in towns, villages or cities in India where tea or coffee is not served to the guests. The publicity in favour of tea and coffee has declared these as antioxidant and they are supposed to kill cancer germs.

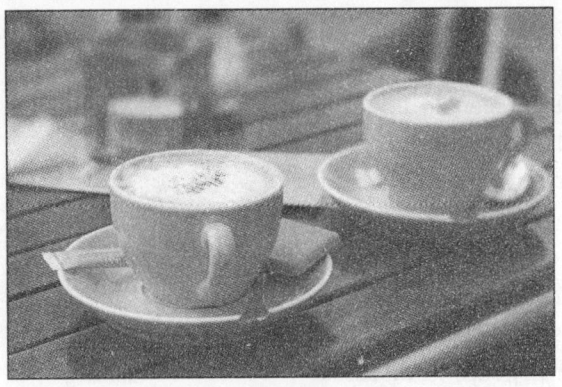

Coffee

In northern India there is a myth that excessive intake of tea darkens the complexion. This is a myth and no harm is done to the complexion by taking two or three cups of tea. Nevertheless, excessive intake of tea and coffee is naturally has bad impact.

BEAUTY BATHS

If you are under impression that cleaning the skin by washing it frequently can improve your complexion, you are wrong. Taking bath has only one benefit on the skin that it gets cleaned and free of dirt. Bathing gives back the original texture of the skin. Apply soap twice a week only. In summer have two baths a day. Wash your hair everyday, if possible but do not apply shampoo every day. Use a body brush for cleaning knees, elbows, ankles, back and calves. Too much application of soaps snatches oily contents of the skin along with dirt.

On the days when you do not use soap, rub your body with your hands or body-brush and go on pouring water to remove the dirt. Wipe your body with a soft towel. This will help activate every cell of the skin become alive with blood due to frictional effect of the towel. Naturally, a good skin has healthy cells. The towel used should be dried under the sun so that no fungus develops. Never wear the clothes without wiping the skin dry by a towel. If you wear clothes on wet skin, it will be like inviting skin rashes and diseases.

Herbal Beauty Bath

Ayurveda brings in the latest facilities in the field of beauty baths. There are many Ayurvedic beauty clinics in India and baths can be taken there. There are three types of baths in their clinics—Oil- baths, Milk-baths and Herbal-baths. Along with these baths, some internal medicines are given in these clinics if the patients are suffering from skin disorders.

Oil-baths

In oil baths, some herbs are mixed and a massage is given to the person desiring the bath. Three persons do it at a time. One person is responsible for keeping the temperature of oil in order and other two apply the oil all over the body. This application and massage goes on for an hour and then herbal body-pack are applied over the oil. After some time, this pack is removed with the help of a cotton cloth.

Milk-bath

Milk bath is not done with pure milk but milk with many herbs, flowers and sandal powder. The person lies down on the table and then milk is poured all over his/her body. Gentle rubbing of body is done while pouring milk for fifteen or twenty minutes. Now a body pack is applied on the whole of body and allowed to dry before the body is showered with plenty of water.

Herbal-bath

This bath is given to the person when he or she has some skin ailments and require attention. General herbal bath is also offered in the clinics. For this, herbal water for this type of bath is made ready one night prior to date of bath. Herbs are put in the water and allowed to stay overnight and then boiled to make one fourth of the total water. The remaining water is then filtered and with this water, the bath is given in a fixed manner as desired by the clinic authorities.

Note: After the bath, it is not essential that you should have the beauty-pack applied. It costs more and so is considered to be exceptional.

Aroma-bath for a Fresh Bath-feeling

Aroma baths or scented baths have their own advantages. They make one feel fresh. In these types of aroma baths, no synthetic scents are added in water but some natural oils or herbs are used, which are very beneficial for the body. These baths are also available in health clinics. If you want to try the pleasure of such baths at home, try this.

Take juice of two oranges and two lemons and mix them. Pour this mixture in a bucket full of water and take a bath. Do not apply soap during this bath. After the bath, do not rub your skin with towel but gently press it dry with soft towel. You will feel very fresh after this bath and the skin will also absorb some vitamins through this bath.

Bath can also be taken after mixing one tablespoon of honey or a bucket of water. Mix some eu-de-colone in the bucket of water to have feeling of freshness in summer.

Eight Enemies of Complexion

- Advancement of age
- Lack of sleep
- Lack of nutritional food
- Alcohol
- Smoking, chewing tobacco
- Lack of exercise
- Exposure to sun and polluted environment
- Wrong life-style

HOME REMEDIES

Though the markets today are flooded with cosmetics not everyone can afford the cost of the same and not everyone can use them due to their reliability and suitability to each one of them. What then remains is the home made product that is harmless and if found not suiting to the individual's skin, the usage can be immediately stopped. Moreover, these home made products have no adverse effects. They are time tested and almost legendary.

Face-cleansing and Masks Formulae

If you are not willing to use soap for cleansing of your body, here are few alternative recipes.

Get dry powdered Indian gooseberry (Amla) and mix coconut oil in it to make a paste. Apply this on the face and the body in place of soap for a fairer complexion.

Rub a mixture of black gram powder mixed with castor oil or if the skin is oily, instead of castor oil, mix water. Make a paste and apply on the face. Keep it at least for ten minutes and then wash it with warm water.

After taking a bath, rinse the face with a mixture of juice of Basil leaf and lemon juice.

A mixture of black gram powder and milk is also a good combination for cleaning the face. Apply the paste of this mixture and let it be there for ten minutes to dry. Rinse it with fresh water. Do it daily.

Make a mixture of two tablespoons of honey, one tablespoon of milk powder, one small tablespoons of limejuice and one-fourth teaspoon of turmeric powder. Make a paste and apply it on the face. Leave it to dry which will take about 15 minutes. Rinse the face with water. Do it once a week.

CARE OF DRY SKIN IN REFERENCE TO COMPLEXION

Do not apply soap over the dry skin. With some barley flour, add some butter and olive oil. Make a paste, apply daily on the face, and let it remain there for ten minutes. Wash the face gently with warm water. Continue this for one month and see the difference.

To add glow to your dry face, grind some yellow lentil or get it ready made from the market. Mix some milk cream in it and make a paste. Apply it on the face and wash the face with warm water after fifteen minutes.

Mix turmeric powder with sandalwood powder and make a paste with olive oil. Apply this paste on your arms, legs, neck and body. After about 15 minutes, take a bath. The skin will have a moisturized look.

Cut and grind some carrots, some cabbage leaves and pieces of radish. Boil the mixture. After boiling, filter the mixture and cool the water. Wash your face with this water and then apply the remains of this vegetable mixture on the face as a mask. Let it be there for 15-20 minutes and then wash the face. This mask is very useful for dry skin. It will improve upon the complexion and make the skin tender.

Milk Cream Combinations for Dry Skin

Add two drops of honey in milk cream and massage with this pack on the face and neck. Let it remain on the face for one hour and then take bath. Milk cream and turmeric powder can also be mixed and applied if honey is not readily available. Do it daily. Milk cream mixed in wheat flour makes a good paste too. Apply this paste on your face except lips, eyebrows and eyes. Bathe after five minutes.

Care of Oily Skin

Take some fuller's earth and add one teaspoonful of honey and two teaspoonful of yogurt. Make a paste, apply on the face for ten minutes, and then wash your face.

Take a ripe tomato. Cut it and grind it in the mixer to make a puree. Add to it a teaspoonful of lemon juice and then mix both of these with barley flour. Make a paste and apply on the face for twenty five minutes or so. This is a very useful paste to extract the extra oil from the face and its regular use improves the complexion.

At least three times a week it should be applied for better results.

Warm a tablespoon full of honey slightly and then add one teaspoon of lemon juice in it. Apply this mixture on the face. After it dries up, wash the face with fresh water.

Mix half to one spoon of sandalwood powder with four or five drops of rose water and the same quantity of milk. Apply this paste on the face. Leave it for about15 minutes and then wash with warm water.

Improving the Complexion of Mixed Skin

Apply ripe papaya pulp on the face. Leave the same on the face for15 to 20 minutes and then wash the face with fresh water.

Take 3 tablespoons of corn flakes. Add one teaspoon of milk, one teaspoon of honey and one teaspoon of the white portion of an egg. Make a paste and apply on the face. Let it be there for 15-20 minutes and then wash the face.

Take one egg and separate its yellow part. Add half teaspoon of honey and one teaspoon of milk powder to it. Mix this mixture thoroughly and then apply this paste on the face. Let it be there for twenty to twenty five minutes and then wash your face.

Improving the Complexion of General Skin

Scrap out some fresh coconut and extract its milk. Apply this milk on the face and lips. This maybe done while retiring to bed.

Take some unboiled milk. Soak a piece of cotton in it and apply the cotton on your skin. Repeat this cleaning procedure with different cotton-pieces. It will clean the skin and make it bright.

Take one cup yogurt. Add one tablespoon of orange juice and the same quantity of lime juice. Make a paste and apply it on the face. After fifteen minutes, clean the face with wet tissue paper slowly.

Make a protein mask to enhance the glow of your face. Take a teaspoon of horsebean and 7 pieces of almonds. Soak them in water for a night. Then grind both of them to make a paste in some water. Apply this paste and keep for 30 minutes and then wash the face. This treatment improves the complexion.

Grind the seed of Jambul (an evergreen tropical fruit) to make a powder. Now mix milk cream in it to make a paste. Apply this paste on the face and let it dry.

When it is dried, wash the face. Do it for 15 days and see the change in your complexion. It will be brighter than before.

Put some turmeric powder in lukewarm milk and drink it daily for an improvement in your complexion.

USE OF SOAPS AND FACE WASHES

We all wash our faces with or without soap. The purpose is to clean it and make it breathe easily. The sparkle of the face is maintained by washing the face. Soaps were considered the best cleaning agents and are used widely in both urban and rural regions.

Face washes have become a necessary tool of cleaning for the people in the cities. Face wash as the name indicates is utilized to clean the face only. For rest of the body, good quality soaps serve the purpose of cleaning. Soap is not a beauty product but a face wash is a beauty product for sure.

Soaps in general have certain types of chemicals that make the skin dry and their constant use takes away the natural oil of the face. Face washes on the other hand are stated to have harmless ingredients. But one has to select a face wash according to the suitability of one's skin. If wrong faces washes are used, there maybe erupt rashes, wrinkles, red spots and itching.

If the face washes are selected correctly, even acne, pimples, or blackheads can be eliminated! Today it is considered by majority that face washes are better than soaps if the face has to be handled carefully.

Face wash is said to be hundred percent soap-free enriched with natural deep cleansers. Every company has its own ingredients like abstracts of grapes, strawberry, raspberry, orange, margosa, holy Basil, rose-petals, milk, almonds, kesar, aloe vera etc. Face wash should be applied on the face in circular motions massaging the face for some time. Lather will be formed after which the face should be washed. There are various types of face washes available in the market that are suitable for dry skin, oily skin and skin with acne or pimples.

Proper use of Face Wash

- Do not use face wash more than twice in a day.
- Do not wash the face with excessive cold or excessive hot water while using face wash.
- Do not rub your face much with face wash if your face has acne/pimples.
- To dry the face after face wash, use a very soft towel or let it get dry on its own.
- For oily skin, select a face wash that has lemon and cucumber besides other ingredients.
- For dry skin, select a face wash that has glycerin and milk cream besides other things.
- For skin which is full of acne/pimples, select a face wash that has cucumber, mint, margosa and basil leaves besides other things.
- For general skin, select a face wash that has fruits

- For sensitive skin, select a face wash according to the advice of dermatologists.

Herbal Water

It is highly recommended that the application of a base is needed before any face wash is used. Beauty experts recommend e use of herbal wash before applying any face wash. Herbal water is a skin toner. It can be prepared at home. In some water put a few petals of rose petals and leaves of mint and let it remain overnight. In the morning, this water is ready for washing the face.

Removing Make-up for Safe Complexion

If you are used to applying make-up (cosmetics) regularly, it is better to clean the entire make-up at night before retiring to bed. The face should not be washed with water or soap. Do not use a face wash or any beauty soaps to remove make-up. If either of this is done, it will damage the skin's complexion.

Make a paste of yogurt and turmeric powder and apply this paste on the face. Leave it for 15 minutes and then wash the face with cold water. If you have no time to prepare this mixture, you can purchase cleansing milk or make-up remover from the market.

Chapter 8

Features that Add Beauty to the Face

CARE OF TEETH

The beauty of face depends upon the beauty of teeth as well. A beautiful set of white, glistening teeth can go a long way to beautify a face. A beautiful smile can charm its onlookers widely. To achieve this sort of smile where teeth should look an addition to beauty, one has to observe certain rules of cleaning of teeth. Care of teeth is essential.

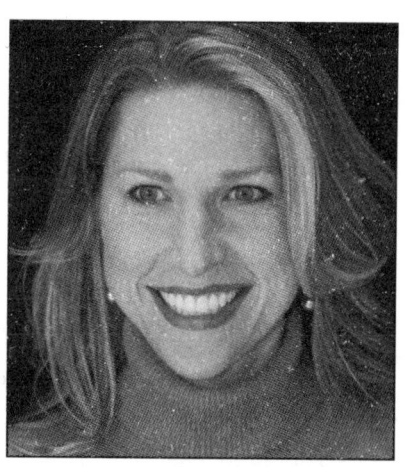

A beautiful smile

Method of Cleaning the Teeth

People from every walk of life know that cleaning of teeth is very essential as dental sepsis and decay occurs. The primary need to keep the teeth and gums healthy is to rinse the mouth and clean the teeth after every meal. Make it a habit. There is a way to brush the teeth also. If the teeth are brushed straight across, the food particles are removed from the outer surface of teeth and not from the spaces between the teeth. Some doctors are of the opinion that teeth should be brushed with a circular motion or with a up and down motion but the practical tests have shown that such a method has some disadvantages. By the up and down motion of the brush, there is a possibility of injuring the gums. The gums will be pushed upward or downward away from the necks of the teeth. In case, a child or an adult is already having very soft gums, or inflamed or loose gums, the food will be brushed under the loose gums, which in turn may give rise to pyorrhoea.

Keeping this in view some doctors are of the opinion that the teeth should be swept by a brush in one direction only. There is another school which opines that the upper teeth should be brushed by sweeping downwards and the lower teeth should be swept with the brush in the upward direction.

Preserving the Health of Teeth

Our ancestors have been practicing the following methods to keep teeth and gums healthy. It is interesting to note that modern methods do not make go into any kind of controversy with these methods since these measures appear to be logical. You may observe these methods for yourself and see why.

Clean the teeth twice a day, early in the morning and then before going to bed.

After taking each meal, rinse your mouth with water for at least ten times. Rinsing is not just putting water in the mouth and throwing it out after circulation but the help of your fingers should be taken for rubbing the gums along with water in the mouth.

When you eat a hot substance, do not take cold water immediately.

Do not take very hot or very cold things.

Use tooth picks after each meals and rinse the mouth after it so that there is no food particle left in it.

If you are having some problems of the teeth, avoid taking pickles which is of acidic nature and may weaken the enamel, particularly at the neck of the teeth.

If you cannot avoid sweets or food containing sugar, say milk, rinse your mouth with water after such an intake. The same stands good for ice creams, and toffees etc.

Do not take tobacco before going to bed. In no case, there should be any such chewable things, even betel nut, while you go to sleep.

Taking bed tea in the morning without brushing or cleaning teeth is bad for teeth. Tea may increase the heat of the body and will increase bile already accumulated during night. The first thing in the morning should be drinking of water instead of tea. Take at least two to three glasses of water in empty stomach. The bed tea may end in hyperacidity in most of the cases.

Finally chew your food properly before swallowing so that indigestion is avoided. Do not take food in haste. You maybe in a hurry but your stomach is never in a hurry to digest it.

Our teeth are not meant for tearing apart substances which are elastic in nature and somewhat hard. This means that our teeth are not shaped or designed to eat non-vegetarian food. Such design and type of teeth are given to such animals, which thrive on flesh of other animals. It has been established practically that people who are basically vegetarians possess more healthy teeth and gums than those belonging to the non-vegetarian group. Try to be strict vegetarians, if the health of your teeth and gums have any significance in your life.

CARE OF NECK

The poets all over the world have praised the beauty of women in many ways and one of the expressions that count much is the beauty of the neck. But with the passage of time and age, the neck muscles show lines and look aged. The strength of the neck muscles become loose.

In some cases, the neck appears darker than the face. It maybe due to the sunrays and hence need treatment under the sunscreen treatment of which we have already discussed.

Irrespective of the size of the neck, be it long, fat or lean, it always need attention and care.

Tips for a Beautiful Neck

The neck is more exposed to the dirt, sun, and pollution. It has to be cared well like the face. The cream you apply on the face should be applied on the neck also after cleaning the neck with wet cotton piece and cleansing lotion.

Similarly, the face pack you apply on the face should be applied on the neck too. Massaging the neck is also very essential while you go to bed. The massage can be done with coconut oil or ghee and the direction of massage should be always in the upward direction.

In the morning some neck exercises should be conducted daily.

Neck Exercises

Take a chair to sit. Keep your back straight on your chair and now look towards right shoulder moving your neck slowly. Keep this posture for a while and now repeat this with change of direction that is, look towards your left shoulder moving the neck slowly. After doing this for two times on both sides, make your neck straight and nod slowly three times. In this process, you chin should touch the chest.

Move your hips forward to the edge of the chair. Sit straight and keep your hands on the rest of chair. Now turn your body to right side as if you are looking behind. Remain in this posture for a while and now do it again turning your body to left side. Do it three times. Slowly move your neck clockwise to make a round. Repeat this for three times. Now move your neck anticlockwise, three times.

CARE OF KNEES, ELBOWS AND ANKLES

If you happen to see the models on a ramp, you might have noticed that they do not have blackish marks on knees, elbows, and ankles. How do they maintain this natural complexion that goes right with the colour of their skin? Every girl and every woman can achieve this provided care is given to this part of the body. The colour of knees, elbows, and ankles become comparatively black when compared with the other skin due to dryness. You may try this and see the result. While taking a bath, regularly scrub these parts of the body with an earthen scrubber or threaded brush or medium-hard plastic brush. All these things are available in big beauty shops.

Apply some good soap and add some lemon to a jug of water, which should be used for washing and scrubbing.

Scrub the parts for about ten minutes and then wash with lemon containing water.

Do not use soaps that contain chemicals. After the bath, apply lacto-calamine lotion on the parts with gentle hand. Do not rub the lotion.

At night while going to bed, wash the parts and soak them dry and then apply the above lotion.

Every week, say on Sundays, when you have time, apply lemon directly on knees, elbows and ankles by cutting it into two pieces. After this apply honey and salt mixed together on the parts with slight pressure massage. Leave the skin to absorb the contents for fifteen minutes and then apply some good moisturizer as prescribed in this book.

Take help of a beauty clinic to use skin tanner. The tanner lotion is available in the market also. Check that these tanners for knees, elbows, and ankles have moisturizers and colour. See that the colour matches your skin and also check that the colour is not in much quantity.

CARE OF HAIR

If there's something that all ladies dreads regarding their appearance that is not the complexion but appearance of their hair. Every woman longs for long, shiny and lustrous hair on the head to enhance her beauty. Since this topic has been dealt with separately in a book named 'Hair Care' authored by me, I shall advise the readers to purchase the book published by B. Jain Publishers, New Delhi for complete guidance. Here I shall reproduce some vital facts about hair that will interest all the readers.

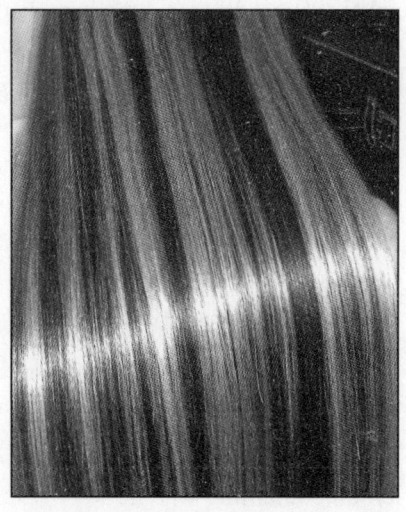
Care of hair

Trichologists and scientists have studied that average human being has 100,000-120,000 hairs on the scalp. A person sheds about one hundred strands of hair everyday on an average. Ninety percent of these falling hairs are 'Anagen' hair and ten percent of these hairs are 'Catagen' or 'Telogen'. (Figures are for healthy individuals on an average) If one opts not to have a hair cut, the hair would achieve a length of about 106 cm and then would fall.

When a lady reaches the age of forty to fifty years, her twenty percent of hair are already fallen. In this hair, the hair becomes dry. In a month the hair grows about 12 mm length of hair.

The speed of hair growing is more during the age of fifteen to twenty five or so. In summer, the hair growth is more than in winter.

During sleep, the hair grows more than when awake. There are many problems concerning the hair but the most visible problem is dandruff. The other problems are caused by diseases which have to be treated but dandruff can be removed at home taking some care as briefed below:

General Causes of Dandruff

- Abrupt change of climate for a person going from cold to hot or hot to cold.
- Wearing a tight scarf or a tight cap or hat. (Some doctors or trichologists do not agree with this).
- Not washing the hair regularly when they are dirty
- Tensions and worries
- Excessive use of hair sprays, gels, colours and dyes.

General Symptoms of Dandruff

- White or yellow flakes that come out when scratched or combing

- Intense itching of scalp
- Acne or pimples on the forehead
- Dry flakes on eyebrows or eyelashes
- White spots on the face

Treatment of Dandruff

To a common man or woman, dandruff is identified when there are flaky dry particles (dead skin) in the hair with an oily sheen. Dandruff arises from oily scalps and not dry scalps. Most of the people think that dandruff can be removed by washing with medicated shampoo available in the market. To some extent it is true. It is said that food that have artificial colours, preservatives of additives should be avoided when dandruff takes place.

The best home method is to give a regular treatment to the hair by massaging the scalp with coconut oil, every night. In the morning, the hair maybe washed with shampoo. Massaging a mixture of coconut oil, Sesame oil and Indian gooseberry oil and washing the hair after one hour of such application removes good lot of dandruff.

Keeping the hair clean is the best method of treatment of dandruff. And for this, you have to shampoo daily as you comb and brush your hair daily. Selection of a suitable shampoo is a must in this case.

Stop using hair styling products on your hair.

Stop using cap and turbans. Wearing such headgears can stimulate the process that is responsible for dandruff.

In case you have purchased an anti-dandruff shampoo, use it once or twice a week and on other days, use regular shampoo that is not meant for dandruff. This will fetch good results.

Some experts say that olive oil mixed with rosemary oil when massaged in the scalp instead of coconut oil gives better results. In this case also the hair should be left overnight before washing them in the morning.

The most common preparation to remove dandruff used to be glycerin and eau-de-cologne. People do not use this mixture now.

Some homoeopathic manufacturing companies have brought in some brands of shampoos claiming that they do not have chemicals. Those brands, if having certain indigenous herbal plants like Reetha, shikakai (ayurvedic herbs) and Amla (Indian gooseberry), should be very useful.

It is said that gentle massaging of table salt on the scalp and leaving the same for fifteen minutes and then washing removes dandruff.

Before washing the hair, massage some vinegar on the scalp and leave it for one hour. Wash the hair now. Repeat this twice or thrice a week.

It is also the frequency of washing the hair that becomes a tool for removing the dandruff. In winter, people wash their hair only once a week thus allowing dust to accumulate in the hairs. This aggravates the condition.

Two tablespoonful of malt vinegar should be dded in a glass having 250 ml of water. Shampoo your air and then rinse the hair with this solution. Dry the hair in the natural way.

Avoid eating fried food, nuts, chocolates, and animal fat.

Take milk and its products, green vegetables, fish, chicken and products that contain Vitamin A, E and B complex.

Two tablespoonfuls of fenugreek seeds should be soaked in water overnight. Next morning, grind the seeds and make a paste.

Apply this paste on the hair and leave them for an hour. Rinse the hair with fresh water using a good herbal shampoo.

Grind four teaspoon of poppy seeds in some milk and apply on the roots of hair. Let it remain on the hair for half an hour and then wash the hair with shampoo. Do this twice a week.

In a cup of yogurt, mix some salt and mix it with little water. Rub the mixture in the hair and then wash the hair after half an hour.

Take four teaspoon of gram flour and make a paste of it in water. Apply this and let it remain for about fifteen minutes. Wash the hair with shampoo.

Two Methods to Remove Dandruff Quickly

1. Warm two teaspoonful of castor oil (quantity according to the length of the hair). Message this lukewarm oil into hair twice or thrice a week at night. Leave the oil overnight and in the morning, wash your hair. Continue this procedure for two weeks and you will find dandruff gone.
2. Dilute some cider vinegar in water and add some lavender oil. Message this oil in the hair every night. Wash your hair in the morning. Do this for seven days and you will find your dandruff gone!

CARE OF LIPS

The expression of love and affection is perhaps best expressed through kissing. And if such is the case, then all ladies should taking good care of their lips. Your face will look good only if the lips on the face are in a healthy state. Some people have problems of dry lips both in winter and summer. You have to protect your lips from the harsh weather conditions. Lips do not have melanin glands that protect the rest of the skin from the harsh effects of the sunrays and hence one has to be careful about the health of the lips.

Lipsticks

Wearing Lipstick is a fashion of the day and it makes lips shining, soft, and colourful. Its quality must suit the skin properties of the lips. It consists of wax, pomade, or cocoa butter, in varying amounts, with either carmine or some aniline dye. It is very rare to see a lipstick wearer having any skin trouble. Where there are splits in the lips, or in rare instances, where absorption of the aniline dye has taken place, serious consequences may result.

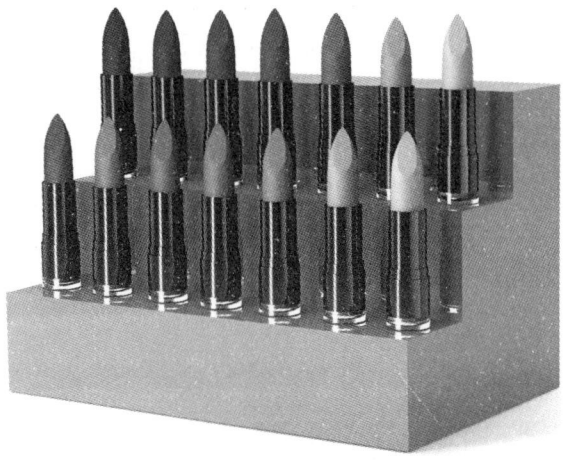

Lipsticks

Home Remedies for Lip Care

Take one teaspoon of glycerin and mix in it half teaspoon of almond oil. This can be used daily on the lips and can be considered a lip-gloss to give shine to the lips.

Mix some lemon juice in two teaspoons of coconut oil and put this mixture in natural wax. Apply this mixture at night to act as a moisturiser.

If the area around your lips is blackish, you can try this. Mix a powder of almonds, powder of sandal and milk in a quantity that makes a paste like lotion. Apply this lotion gently around the lips for many days continuously at the time of going to bed.

If the lips are blackish, use salt with some milk as a rub on the lips for some days. Do not rub harshly or there will be cuts on the lips. Rub the mixture gently before taking a bath and clean it with water after some time.

Lip-stains

In the market there is liquid lipstick available and it is not the same as lip-gloss. It is called lip-stains in liquid form or tablets with an applicator sponge or brush. It is more of oil than wax.

Lip Crayons and Pencils

Lip crayon is like pencil but has silky touch and is more malleable for use as a replacement of lipsticks. Pencils are like regular pencils that can be evenly sharpened. The application can be artistic and can be thick or thin at places as desired on the lips.

Lip-gloss

The women who are in service and remain out of home for several hours should use lip-gloss on the lips. It is basically meant to give a shining look, youthful appeal to the lips. Lip-gloss is available in dip-in bottle, tubes and tablets. You may also use a lip liner in summer, as this will prevent flowing of the lip-gloss from the lips. This condition is only found in summer days. Lip-gloss covering can also be given after application of lipstick. Before purchasing lip-gloss from the market, be sure to see that it has SPF of 15 that is ideal for summer. Lip-gloss with SPF-

15 protects lips against ultra-violet rays of the sun and gives a good protection to the lips from getting darkened. (For details about SPF, see page 47 under caption SPF factor and sunscreen)

Proper Use of Lipsticks and Lip-gloss

- To be on the safer side, apply glycerin or lip balm on the lips before going to bed at night especially in winter.
- Use only good quality lipsticks so that cheap chemicals do not harm the texture of the lips.
- To avoid the cracking of lips and the dry condition, apply mustard oil on the naval every day after taking bath. Take vitamin 'E' on the prescription of doctor, if allowed.
- Eat plenty of green vegetables and fruits.
- Take sufficient water.
- Apply lip-gloss or balm to keep lips moisturised.
- While purchasing lipsticks, test the colour or shade of the item on your finger-tips and not on the back of hand. Lips and finger tips have the same texture to test colour of lipsticks when you can not apply the product on your lips.
- Do not use lipsticks that have expired in their validity. Never use lipsticks that are two years old.

Homoeopathic Treatment for Lip Ulcers

If there are ulcers on the lips, behind the lips or around the lips, they mar of the beauty of face. To treat this, you have to consult a homoeopath for quick relief.

There are few suggestions for remedies you can use:
Pain inside lips: Calc. sulph.

Lower lip, inner surface: Phos.

Lower lip, inner left side: Ars. M.

Upper lip: Caust., Staph., Zinc., Merc. sol., Kali carb., Mez.

Lower lip
Caust., Clem., Ign., Lyco., Phos., Sepia, Silicea, Sulph., Zinc.

Corners of lips
Amm.mur., Bell., Borax, Calc. carb., Hep sulph., Graph., Merc sol., Nat mur., Nit acid., Rhus tox, Sil., Staph., Sul.

Note: Do not take these medicines without the guidance of a homoeopath.

KAJAL FOR YOUR EYES

In India, the importance of kajal (a black lining given all around the eyes) is known to young girls right from their childhood. Application of kajal makes the eyes look broader and bigger. It is a traditional act for in the Indian culture to make kajal at home. But this is in the rural areas. In the urban areas, it is available with the shopkeepers under many branded names. In Europe of USA, it is not common to use kajal in the eyes and in place the eyeliner is used. The eye-specialists in India do not recommend the application of kajal in the eyes of kids.

Making Kajal at Home

In an earthen lamp, put some ghee (a fatty substance) and insert a cotton wick over the edge of lamp. Mix some camphor in it. Now light the lamp. Put an inverted metal spoon over the flame of lamp. The carbon formed on the surface of the spoon is kajal. Now scratch this carbon with your finger from the spoon's surface and add ghee. This is kajal ready for application.

Kajal is also made with the help of almond oil, and mustard oil in place of ghee with or without the addition of camphor.

CARE OF THE BACK

It is seen that women greatly take care of face and forget to pay attention to hands, feet, neck, elbows, heels, and back. The back should also be made target of attention. The exposed area of the neck and back is visible to the eyes of people and if these areas are neglected, the whole of the beauty of the face becomes a waste.

Methods to Clean the Back

Beauty experts emphasize scrubbing of the back. The dead skin of the back is removed by scrubbing and in its place comes the fresh glowing skin. When the neck and the exposed back is open to sun, the area gets affected and becomes black. If one does not want this situation, it is better to cover the neck and back when going out in the sun. It is still better to use umbrella so that the parts are not exposed to the sun. While taking a bath, the back and neck should be cleaned with the help of a handle-brush available in the market. If the skin of your back is thick in texture, do not wear wide opening blouses.

In winter, the dry cold winds make the skin dry. The normal moisture in the skin gets faded. One should use moisturiser on the back. After the bath, it is better to apply body lotion and moisturiser on the back and neck so that the skin does not get dry sooner. In the market, accessories for cleaning of the back are available. This includes brushes with long handle and 'Lufa'. Lufa is made of either plastic of scrub material (plant scrub that is used to clean heels). It is a long stretchable bandage that has two handles to insert your hands.

USES OF BRUSHES

There are many types of brushes available in the beauty shops. These brushes are used in applying various types of make-up.

These are fully utilized by the beauty parlours. At home also, these can be used but one should know the typical function of each brush. Some of the brushes are:

- *Liner brush:* This is used to draw lines on the edges of eyes
- *Eye-shadow brush:* It is used to draw/spread the colours of eye-shadow colouron the upper lids of eyes
- *Eye-gromer (blacken with grime) brush:* It is used to colour the eyelashes and the eyebrows.
- *Lip-liner brush:* As the name indicates, it is for drawing the outer- lines of lips.
- *Lip brush:* This is to spread the lipstick colour on the lips.
- *Foundation brush:* This is used to apply waterproof base foundation on the face.
- *Bindi brush:* As the name suggests, it is to draw Bindi (a mark on the forehead done for beautification) on the forehead especially if the Bindi is to look artistic.

Chapter 9

Medical Help for Beauty

Search for a youthful and attractive appearance has been on the agenda of women since many ages. Manufacturing companies dealing in beauty products are always busy introducing new products. They go to any extent. Claims of converting darker complexion into fairer one is a recent claim. Such claims are not confined to females only but has now extended to the males also. The curious phenomenon is that no advertisements say that a healthy life style and a good diet should also be adhered to with the use of products they claim to promote fair complexion. It is amazing to note that even those who doubt about the claims go in for trial and purchase such types of creams.

The new era of awareness for beauty has come from Europe and United States. Special mention maybe made of a US based research company called the Freedonia group, manufacturer of beauty products has estimated that by the end of 2008, sales of 'appearance-enhancing' supplements will have sale of 2.5 billion dollars! I do not say that claims of giving a fairer skin always fail. There are persons who think they are dark complexioned but are not actually dark. Their dark complexion is due to certain skin diseases and when this skin disease is cured with the use of a beauty product, they get convinced that they have become fair-complexioned.

I have met many Dermatologists and wanted to know whether they recommend such products that claim to make dark complexion fair. No one agreed that any cream or lotion could change the complexion of a person. They do not prescribe such products for their patients. We do have in the market creams and lotions or face packs that contain anti-oxidants or mineral supplements like vitamin C or zinc to make the skin vibrant with health. This is in addition to the old traditional recipe like fish oil. Fish oil has been considered good for the glow of the skin.

Many people often ask whether it is true that beauty products help achieve beautiful skin?

According to many beauty saloons, no pills or supplements can alone promise the betterment of skin. It is local treatment and care of skin that gives the glow to the skin. According to dermatologists vitamin B fights against dry and flaky skin, vitamin A is for skin upkeep and repair, iron, proteins, calcium, folic acid, and vitamin E repairs the skin. Vitamin C helps build collagen that is one of the natural binding ingredients of the skin.

WHAT IS 'BOTOX'?

Botox is the brand name of botulinum toxin type 'A'. It is a protein extracted from bacterium clostridium botulinum marketed by Allergan. There is also a cheap quality of botox called Dysport, which is available in India. Botox and Dysport both are used widely in India for non-cosmetic purposes. Allergan's botox is an injection and sold in vials. It is basically used to erase the wrinkles of the face. These wrinkles can be in the forehead region (horizontal lines and frown lines), Crow's feet (laugh lines running from nasal sides to the chin along the corners of the mouth and bunny lines. In the young and middle age, these wrinkles mostly appear when a person expresses his/her emotions or laughs. Botox is injected into static wrinkles.

'Botox' injections sometimes bring harmful results', says a noted cosmetic surgeon. 'It may lead to the paralysis of face'. On the other hand, most of cosmetic surgeons oppose this view saying that experienced surgeons will never let this happen.

Side Effects of Botox

If the botox is injected in the wrong muscles or given in a wrong dose or in a non-sterile atmosphere, some complications are expected. These are drooping eyelids, difficult chewing if injected in wrong muscle in the jaws, difficult swallowing if injected at different muscles of neck and raised eyebrows if injected wrongly on the forehead muscles. The major side effect of a wrong dose or in wrong muscle is that the face will look dead without any expression.

There are many 'Botox' clinics and organisations looking after this aspect in the world. According to Dr Braun, who runs the biggest 'Botox' clinic in Canada says Botox softens the appearance of any wrinkles.

There is a Cosmetic Physicians Society of Australia studying the improvement on cosmetic surgery. (Courtesy: Mail Today-March 15, 2008). In India we have private clinics run by dermatologists and there are cosmetic surgeons attached to good hospitals.

However, it is a fact that Botox is the most popular method of erasing wrinkles of the face and the neck. The rich and affluent people including film actors are utilizing the wonders of cosmetic surgery and trying to remain young in their looks.

Chapter 10

Nails

Nails are a very important part of a woman's overall beauty. The beauty of nails earlier was a concern of women but now males are also conscious about the look of their nails. They are now getting their nails manicured. Every part of the human body has some purpose for which it is made. Nails in the body have a purpose also. In this modern fast moving world, decoration and upkeep of nails is an upcoming profession in the health and beauty industry. This is because beautiful nails on fingers or toes deserve appreciation only if they are healthy, decorated, well-groomed, nicely trimmed, shaped and polished. Cosmetic care of nails is called manicure. Nails are integral ornaments of the body.

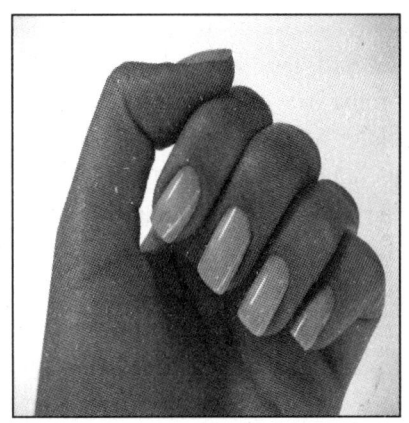

Trimmed nails look neat

HOW ARE NAILS RELATED WITH THE BODY?

Nails are embedded into the skin from three sides. It is the skin that holds the nail. Skin is the outer layer of the body that has complex and multiple uses. In whole of the body, there is no other organ that has varied duties to perform as the skin again, which is constantly subjected to outside exposures and injuries. The functions of the skin are very essential for life. If the skin is destroyed near the tips of fingers, it will not be able to hold the nail in its place. Protection of skin around nails is important because of the fact that it is this skin that has to protect the nails, regulate heat or cold around the nails and fully appreciate the sensations around the nails.

Every person has a different size in case of nail plates. This individual difference is hereditary. The average length of a nail plate is 10 to 15 mm; its width is from 10 to 17 mm while its thickness varies from 0.30 to 0.37 mm. There is a variation in the sizes of nail plates of both hands. It is due to exerting of pressure on the working hand. As the baby is born, it has same size of nail plates on both hands but as the baby grows and starts working with its hands, pressuring the fingers and nails, the working hand gets the impact of work and the width of the nail plate gets flattened or widened. If the person is working with the right hand, his right hand nail plate will be wider than the left hand nail plate. If the person is a left-hander and performs all his works with the left hand, his left hand nail plates will be wider than right hand nail plates. Growth of nails is different from the growth of hair. The growth of nail is a continuous process and without any definite limit. It also depends from person to person, his or her occupation and the general state of health. In warm weather, the growth of nail is more as compared to the people living in cold weather. Growth of nail is also more in youth than in old age. With the advancement of age as the body gets weaker and has no other growths, the growth of nails also becomes slower.

In men, nails grow faster than in women. For a right-hander, the nails on the right hand grow faster than the left hand and for a left-hander; nails grow faster on the left hand than the right hand. It has been estimated that it requires from one hundred to one hundred sixty days for an entire fingernail to grow. Some doctors are of the opinion that it takes 96 to 115 days for the complete renewal of the nail. Some doctors have worked out that it takes 100-160 days to reproduce an entire finger nail. The toenail growth takes more time and it is about three times more than the period required for the fingernail for reproduction of entire toenail. The toenails growth rate is about two to three times less than the growth rate of finger nails.

DISEASES AND NAILS

Yours nails will never look beautiful, if you have some disease of nails. The following are common causes of nails getting disordered:

- Lack of cleanliness
- Unrestrained growth (in the case of bedridden or aged patients through neglect of the attendants) Constant pressure of ill-fitting shoes
- Accidents and traumas
- Rheumatism and gout
- Chronic bone diseases
- Degenerative or irritative neuroses
- Chronic inflammatory processes of the skin, which include eczema, syphilis, leprosy, psoriasis, felon, lichen rubber, elephantiasis tuberculosis and occupational dermatoses.
- If you have any one of above disorders or you are not cleaning your nails in time, better consult a doctor.

NAIL BITING

Biting nails or nails or nibbling is a habit with children and adults which have a great bearing with hangnails. When you bite your nails, you also bite the cuticles along the sides and bottom of your nails. This is how hangnails are developed. Once the hangnails are developed, you bite these hangnails with your teeth. This sort of peeling the hangnails by pulling and ripping action of teeth cause development of more of hangnails. The nail biting has to be stopped if you want to avoid hangnails and make them beautiful.

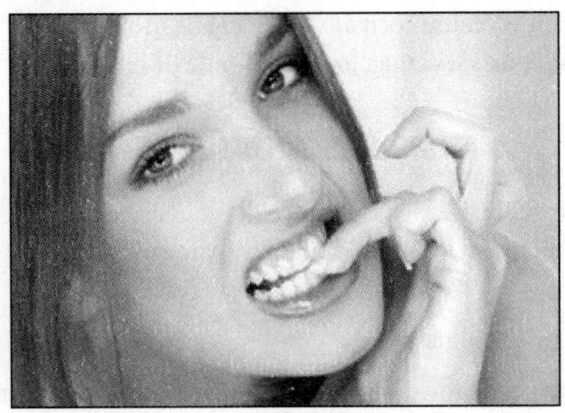

Nail biting

If the nail polish used on the nails is quick-drying, it can also dry the cuticles and cause hangnails. Such quick-drying nails polishes should be avoided. Inferior quality of nail polish should not be used.

Enhancing the beauty of nails with diet and food. The nails can be treated well at home y means of corrected diet and food.

Here are a few tips:
- Those who are prone to nail affections time and again, they should take care of their diet.
- If the nails are splitting and breaking, vitamin A deficiency

maybe there. Carrot, eggs and milk should be taken in such cases.

- For bacterial or fungal infections, it is better to increase intake of onions and garlic along with increase of green leafy vegetables.
- The food we take, has a great role in bringing nail affections and treating them as well. We have many herbs, food items, vegetables, and fruits that cure nails with problems. Their intake and application has been found effective in nails affections.

Food Items that Help in Nail Affection

If a part of a nail has been broken by some injury and is painful, leaves of pomegranate should be grinded and a paste of the same be made with little water. This should be applied on the broken nail.

If the nails are dry and lack shine, immerse the nails in a lukewarm castor oil for sometime everyday. The oil need not be thrown and can be used everyday after heating it. Repeat this immersion act of nails for about seven days. If you cannot do this, apply castor oil on the nails with some cotton every night before retiring. Alternatively, application of glycerin with the help of cotton on the nails will also serve the purpose to remove dryness and bring shine on the nails.

If there is slow growth of nails, squeeze some lemon juice in warm water, immerse fingers in it for five to seven minutes, and then put your fingers in cold water. Repeat this three times and continue this treatment for about seven days. There is another method also. Lemon cut into two parts, can be rubbed against each tip of fingers and around the nails. After rubbing the juice of lemon in this way, allow the fingers to dry and then wash the fingers after about ten minutes.

For making the nails strong, apply coconut oil on the nails and the tips of fingers daily.

Beautiful Nails with Massage and Exercise

Massage of the body of the swollen or painful part of the body has been in vogue since times immemorial. A massage of the hair after a haircut, a massage of the legs with some oil after tiredness, athletic events and long walks is a blessing to the body's health. Massaging and the exercise of fingers in particular has a beneficial effect on the nails. If you happen to see the nails of a musician who plays a 'harmonium', 'sitar', 'tabla' or any other instrument that needs the help of fingers, you will find that their nails are mostly free of diseases.

Similarly, typing work on a typewriter or a computer for some time in a day is a good exercise for keeping the nails healthy. Besides this, there are few exercises that are helpful.

Exercises for Healthy Nails

With the help of right hand thumb and right hand index finger, hold the thumb of the left hand in such a way that your right hand thumb holds the nail bed and the right hand index finger placed exactly beneath the left hand thumb. Now exert slight pressure and release it after counting ten. Repeat it three times. Now hold the index, middle, ring and little fingers of the left hand turn by turn and repeat the same exercise. After the left hand fingers are done with, you can now hold the right hand fingers turn by turn with your left hand thumb and the index finger and repeat the exercise. Indirectly, you are first making the nail bed pale and then releasing the pressure making it red.

With the help of your right hand index finger, press the tip of the left hand thumb in the direction against the nail growth, count ten and release the pressure. Repeat the same on the other fingers of the right hand. Now with the help of the left hand index finger, press the fingers of the right hand turn by turn in the same manner.

This sort of ischaemia (temporary deficiency of blood) and hyperemia (excessive blood) restores the normal blood circulation in both the above exercises.

Place the left hand on the table, palms facing the table and spread the fingers. Now with the help of the right hand index finger, press the area near the growth of nail for some time and release the pressure. Massage the area with soft strokes of finger near the nail growth junction and the massage should be towards the tip of the finger. Repeat this procedure of action on every finger of your hands.

Massage the areas on both the left and the right lateral walls of the nail. Hold the left hand thumb with the right hand thumb and the index finger at the lateral walls of nail and stroke it outwards with the tip of the thumb while keeping the pressure towards the centre of the nail. Repeat this act with all the fingers.

Fold both your hands in such a fashion (making half-open fist) that the nails of both the hands (except thumbs nails) touch each other. The nails in this way will be in one row. Now rub the nails of all the eight fingers of both hands together in vertical strokes gently. Do it for fifty times. This type of rubbing stimulates the blood in the fingers and according to Su Jok therapy, it improves the overall health of a person.

Scratch the nails turn by turn with the help of thumb. The scratching should be both vertical and horizontal.

Tapping the tips of the fingers gently on the table every day for some time helps in the treatment of chronic disorders of nails. (Su Jok therapy).

Care of Nails

Nails have to be cared for maintaining their beautiful looks. Have the following checks:

Finger Rings

People who have long standing diseases of nails should check the rings in the fingers and toes. If they are ill fitting and press the fingers, the nails will be diseased due to less blood circulation. In case of any numbness of a finger or white spots on the nails, occurs remove the ring for some days and check the results before consulting a doctor.

Check Your Shoes

If your toenails have fungus, or there is itching/disfigurement in the shape of the nails, do not wear plastic shoes. Wear those shoes through which air can pass freely. Select those shoes, which are broad at the toes and there is no squeezing of the toes. Ill-fitting shoes can result in corns on the soles or toes. Better wear socks in the rainy season while jogging or doing exercises. Check your nail polish too.

Nail Polish

If the continuous use of a particular brand of nail polish develops some nail-disease, stop using the same. Change the brand of nail polish. Sometimes change of colour of the nail polish also matters. Each colour belongs to prolonged stimulation methods. According to the colour therapy, there are certain amounts of waves and frequencies that affect the body. Each organ of the body corresponds to a particular frequency. If the frequency of colour coincides with the frequency of the body, nails become full of energy and remain healthy. It is better to use light colours on nails.

How to Apply Nail Polish?

- Insert small pieces of cotton in between the fingers/toes so that the nail polish does not smear the skin.
- Apply the nail polish properly on the entire nail.
- When it dries up, apply the second coat of polish.
- When this also dries up, make a final coating of nail polish.
- With this method of nail polish application, the nail will not look pale and the polish will not spread on the toes.

How to Avoid Pale Nails?

Pale nails are due to anaemic condition. Take enough of milk and milk products. If you are a non-vegetarian, take one egg everyday. Take food items that are rich in vitamin D. Consult a doctor.

Nail-culture Treatment (artificial nails)

Persons having weak and brittle nails can go in for nail culture treatment from professional beauty experts. If the nails are small, broken, having lines, nail culture is highly recommended. This method replaces the nail and an artificial nail is implanted. These cultured nails are as good as the original nails.

Pedicure

Pedicure is a procedure by which you take care of your feet, toes, and nails. In general, women are quite conscious about cleaning their feet and soles in particular though this is not all that is needed.

The feet should appear very attractive. The poets and artists have adored the beauty of nails and feet. Women and girls do not take care of feet and nails regularly. Whenever they are required to go to marriages or parties, they think of a pedicure. In beauty parlours, there are pedicure machines, which remove the dead skin of the feet. Vibrators are used for a massage. There are four methods of pedicure normal, French, deluxe and paraffin. This is better done at parlours. The benefit of pedicure is that nails are not diseased and they remain bacteria free. The tiredness and swelling of the feet is also controlled if it is due to walking and hanging of the feet during traveling.

Pedicure at Home

In case you have no time to get the pedicure done in parlours, here is home-tested method.

- Remove the nail polish of the nails.
- Take some luke warm water in a tub. Add some ammonia, hydrogen peroxide, Dettol and shampoo in it. Some salt can also be added if you are tired.
- Apply cuticle cream to the nails and put your feet in the tub water for ten to fifteen minutes.
- When the water gets a little cold, rub your soles and heels with a scrubber or a pumice stone.
- Clean the nails by a nail brush.
- Massage the nails and toes with cuticle cream.
- Trim your nails with nail cutter and file them with a filer.
- Apply nail polish.

Decorating Toe Nails and Finger Nails

- If your nails are short, you can insert artificial nails by means of glue, available in the market.
- You can apply nail polish according to the colour of the dress you are wearing.

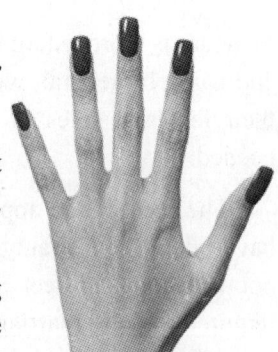
Hands with nail polish

- You can also polish each nail with different colours by vertical or horizontal strokes.

Nail Art and Designs

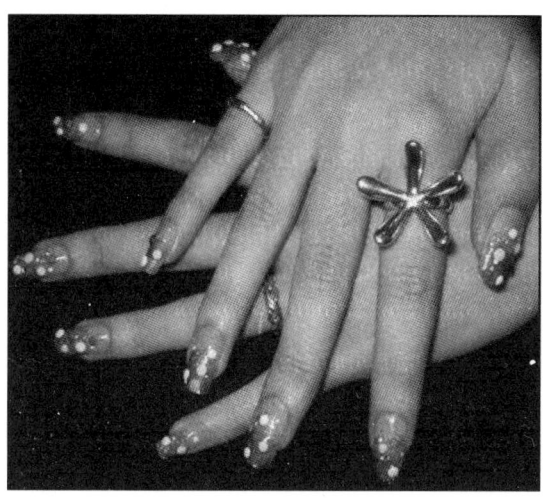

Nail art and nail designs

Nail art and designs is the latest thing available in the world of make-up. It is generally begun with a nice manicure and then the stylist works on a trendy and aesthetic design with paint. Funky nail designs with gold, silver, red, blue, green and black are preferred these days. Many prefer bold colours. Apart from colours, natural hand painting, nail accessorizing, nail piercing, and other innovative things are done on the nails these days.

Note: For complete care of nails, please read my book 'Nail Care' published by M/s B. Jain Publishers, New Delhi.

Chapter 11

Nine Problems of the Face

We all know that diseases and disorders of skin require the help of dermatologist but the occurrence of skin disorders can be handled through domestic measures and means also. Here we shall take up nine most common disorders turn by turn in the following order:

- Acne
- Blackheads
- Blemishes
- Chloasma
- Dark circles around and beneath eyes
- Freckles
- Liver spots
- Moles
- Warts

ACNE AND PIMPLES

Acne is a skin eruption that develops during the period of adolescence and it affects the face, shoulders, chest and the back. Mostly it is confined to the period of adolescence but may attack beyond the age of twenty also. After twenty years of age, the eruption is generally regressed and thereafter it slowly disappears.

The people then experience the presence of scars, which are the results of deep-seated pustules. In course of time, the scars or 'pitting' as it is called, go on vanishing and are less obvious because they formulate the skin in such a way that the whole of the texture of skin looks alike. Acne is more severe in boys than in girls. I treated patients mostly females in the age group of 18 to 20 years who had acne on the chin area and near the corners of the mouth. The rest of the face was clear of any eruptions. This is a typical class of acne that comes for two or three years between 18 to 20 years of age in girls and difficult to treat in a short period. Homoeopathic treatment in such cases has been proved to be very beneficial.

Many women and girls are of the view that acne is due to the inadequate cleaning of the face. This is not true. Acne maybe due to eating a lot of fried, oily and spicy food and chocolates and sweets and nursing lot of tensions on petty matters. Some doctors do not agree to this theory of intake of such types of food and blame hormonal imbalance for acne.

Causes of Acne

Acne or eruptions on a face is a result of physiological adjustment of the skin to the adult state when the whole of body is under the great impact of endocrine glands (Gonads in particular). The result is that the *sebaceous glands get activated with lot of secretions due to their enlarged size. The eruption or acne is the result of uneven adjustments between the anatomical and physiological state of glands during the period of transition. This unequal adjustment moderately obstructs the outflow of sebum. Sebum is retained in the follicle mouth to become imprisoned. This retained and imprisoned sebum increases in amount and the epidermal cells go on adding to it. This takes the shape over the surface of the skin like the leaves of onions and finally results in comedo or blackhead. The other reason stated to be one of the prime reasons is sensitiveness to the normal level of sex hormones. This over sensitiveness produces high level of sebum (oily secretions) that finally ends in acne as stated earlier. (*Sebaceous glands are minute glands in the skin secreting sebum. Sebum is a lubricating substance. Sebaceous glands directly open on the skin. Scalp, face and anus have numerous such glands. Palms and soles are devoid of it.)

In acne, the skin has scattered blackheads or comedones that are more of less numerous. It maybe papules and pustules and in their centre is blackhead. Acne may appear in successive crops. The preferable skin for acne to erupt is mostly oily, greasy and has a flabby appearance. The intensity of the eruptions is variable in different individuals. Acne notifies pimples on the face, neck, shoulders or back. It is eruption of pastular, follicular, or popular type in which sebaceous (oil producing) gland is involved. Its effect comes with the onset of adolescence. Teenagers are the victims of this disorder and the boys are more prone to it than girls. Acne brings in a sort of inferiority complex or distress to the holder but does not cause any serious harm to the health.

Prognosis

The acne can be treated if it is done systematically and persistently. The duration of the treatment depends upon the reasons of acne in particular case and the underlying factors. The individual having acne must have patience and change his or her life style, diet and the routine of life as advised by the doctor. If neglected, acne results in scarring and pitting on the face.

Treatment, General and Domestic

The external treatment of acne is absolutely necessary to ensure that the area affected on the face or body remains clean. Every effort should be made to see that no dirt is accumulated over the eruptions and it is not greasy. No harsh creams or cosmetics should be applied over the acne and doctor's advice should be taken for local applicants. It is better that no cosmetics should be applied. (Homoeopathic view)

Tips

- For cleaning the area of eruptions, simple soap and hot water or fresh water should be used. The soap should be oil free and have solvent quality.

- Boric acid lotion with equal parts of alcohol mixed in it, is a good cleansing agent for acne and this can be used infrequently before going to bed at night.

- The cleansing agents applied at night will subside any irritation on the skin, if any, before morning.

- A lot of 'salad' with meals, more of milk, yogurt and butter help lessen acne.

- Washing the face with oil-free soap after returning home from outside is helpful.

- Avoid more of perspiration by avoiding hot spicy food, junk food and cold drinks.

- Take eatables having more of vitamin A (milk, butter, eggs etc.). Do not take these items in excess. Avoid taking non-vegetarian foods.

- Wash the face at least five times a day.
- Take some gram flour. Mix in it one-fourth teaspoon of turmeric powder and one teaspoon of lemon juice. Keep this mixture aside. Now apply some good quality facial cream (for dry skin) on the face and give the face a massage for about fifteen minutes. Boil some water in a vessel and over it place your face to have steam for some time. Now take pieces of cotton, remove the cream, and clean the face dry. Take the gram flour mixture that had been prepared and kept aside. Apply this mixture on the face and let it be there till it dries. Finally wash the face with fresh water.
- The juice of bitter gourd or cut-pieces of it can be applied on the acne daily while retiring to bed during summer.
- The peels of oranges should be applied on the acne.
- Grind leaves of margosa and mix with a little yogurt. Apply the paste on the acne.
- Juice of one apple mixed with one teaspoon of honey should be applied over the whole of face first and then after 15 minutes, the face should be washed. Apply the same mixture over the acne again. Let it dry and then wash.
- The juice of leaves of mint should be applied on the acne and after it is dried, the face should be washed.

Homoeopathic Treatment at Home

Acne of boys Calcarea picrata 200 One dose daily for 7 days.

Acne of girls Calcarea phos 200, one dose daily for 7 days. At puberty, acne with itching Asterias rub 30

When Astrias rub 30 fails, and eruptions are pustular Kali brom 30, three times a day for 7 days

Pimples with constipation, pimples worse from bath

Magnesia mur 30, three times a day for 7 days Acne on nose

Causticum 30, three times a day for 7 days

Acne on forehead Ledum 30, three times a day for 7 days

Pimples are hard Agaricus 30, three times a day for 7 days

Pimples are moist, digestion slow, flatulence (gas) Carbo veg 30

Rosy pimples, pale skin and chilly feeling Silicea 30

During menses, acne is more and it is harmful to eat sugar, fats, meat, heavy meals, tea and coffee etc. Psorinum 200 weekly one dose, total 3 doses Acne worse in summer Antim crudum 30, three times a day for 7 days.

Note: The dose is of four pills no. 30. If there is no improvement or some improvement, in the above-prescribed period, you must consult a homoeopathic doctor. Also tell the doctor which medicine you had taken, for how many days and whether you were benefited or not.

Cautions for Acne

Do not use cleansers, cold creams or sunscreens having cream base, lotions etc. while treating the acne.

Do not pick or scratch the acne with your nails or fingers. The eruption may aggravate.

Do not use any kind of medicated soap, cream, cosmetics, or lotion without the guidance of a dermatologist. When some creams are prescribed, please see the expiry date of the cream before using. An expired chemical ointment or cream may damage the face.

Drink enough quantity of water; take fruits and green vegetables with nutritional food. Such a routine detoxifies the body.

If you have acne on the back, better wear cotton clothes and avoid use of polyesters or silky garments. Change your clothes everyday.

BLACKHEADS (COMEDONES)

Blackhead is a common disorder of sebaceous function. Small plugs of sebum that fill the gland orifices characterize it. Black colour of the eruption can be white also and they are then called whiteheads. (*Sebaceous glands are minute glands in the skin secreting sebum. Sebum is a lubricating substance. Sebaceous glands directly open on the skin. Scalp, face, and anus are having numerous glands. Palms and soles are devoid of it.)

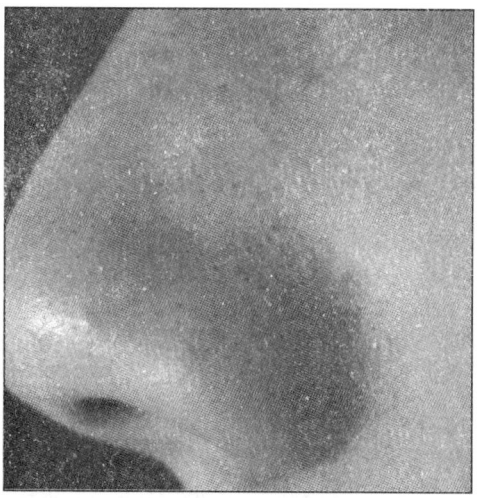

Blackheads

Blackheads are pointed like pins and their size varies from pinpoint to pinhead. These dots of dark green, blackish, or yellow generally are elevated from the facial skin. In many cases these are at a level with the skin and in other cases even below the skin that is, beneath the surface of skin. Generally these are black and hence called blackheads. Girls and boys generally pick them out because they are easily pressed out of the ducts. If they are of recent origin and soft, long thread like filament comes out but the sebaceous matter is firm and it is there beneath the skin. The blackheads have a fatty matter or mass that consists of sebum, epithelial and other debris and microorganisms. The face is not the only location where blackheads are common but they are on the neck, back, and penis. Blackheads maybe very few and or many aggregated or scattered but emit no subjective symptoms. They follow a chronic course with no effect upon the adjoining tissues.

Reasons

They appear due to general or reflex influences arising from acne, gastrointestinal disorders, menstrual irregularities. They are common from puberty to the age of thirty years when glandular and pilary growth is very active. Blackheads are also products of those who are frequently exposed to heat and moisture. People who work in mines, coal dealing, brass, and copper industry, soap factory or water-purifying industry are more prone to blackheads and acne. Blackheads affect both males and females.

Prognosis

Blackheads on the unexposed parts of skin and not subject to irritation need no local treatment because they tend to disappear spontaneously or from general treatment. Actually prognosis primarily depends upon how the patient dealt with them. If he or she is in habit of plucking the blackhead out, the disfigurement of plucked area happens. In this case the help of a medical practitioner is needed. There are blackhead extractors available in beauty clinics and this job should be done from them. The affected surface of blackheads is sponged with glycerin, oil of eucalyptus and rose water. After this a comedo-extractor is employed. The sponging of the face is now done with ready-made lotions. This procedure is repeated every week or even twice a week till the visible blackheads are clear. Out of these removed blackheads, a few will re-form and few new may come up. This means a course of few months is needed for the complete removal of blackheads.

Remedies from the Kitchen

Instead of the exfoliation scrub available in the market one can easily do this with materials from the kitchen. Take sugar and salt in equal quantity and mix them. Now take rose water and mix in sugar and salt so as to make a paste. Apply this paste on the blackheads and give a gentle massage over them for 15 to 20 minutes. Wash the face.

Cut a raw potato in a round shape and rub the same on the blackheads. Then keep the piece on the blackhead for some time. Wash the face.

The juice of a bitter gourd or pieces cut out of it can be applied on the acne daily while retiring for bed during summer.

The skin of oranges should be applied on the acne.

Take one teaspoonful powder of dried skin of oranges, one teaspoon of orange juice, two teaspoon of holy basil leaves juice, two or three flakes of saffron, five to ten drops of rose water and mix them. Massage your face and blackheads in particular for fifteen to twenty minutes with this mixture. Then wash the face.

Grind leaves of margosa and mix with yogurt. Apply the paste on the acne. Juice of one apple mixed with one teaspoon of honey should be applied over the whole of face first and then after 15 minutes, the face should be washed. Now apply the same mixture again over the acne. Let it dry and then wash.

Apply the juice of garlic on the blackheads several times a day. After each application of two or three minutes, wash the area.

Dry some lemon tree leaves and grind it into powder. Mix

turmeric powder in equal quantity. Make a paste and apply on the blackheads. Leave the paste for ten to fifteen minutes and then wash the face.

Take one teaspoon of sandalwood powder, one-fourth teaspoon of coconut water and few drops of lemon juice. Mix them to make a paste and apply on the blackheads. Leave the paste there till it is dry. Wash the face.

Make a paste of one teaspoon of sandalwood powder and one teaspoon of powdered seeds of mustard in some water. Apply the paste on blackheads and let it dry. Afterwards wash the face.

Homeopathic Treatment of Black/White Heads

Blackheads of boys—Calcarea Picrata 200 one dose daily for 7 days.

Blackheads of girls—Calcarea Phos 200 one dose daily for 7 days.

At puberty, acne with itching, Astrias rub 30. When strias rub 30 fails, and eruptions are pustular Kali brom 30 should be used, three times a day for 7 days.

Blackheads on nose—Causticum 30, three times a day for 7 days

Blackheads on forehead—Ledum 30 for 7 days

Blackheads are very hard Agaricus 30, 7 days

Blackheads soft, digestion slow, flatulence (gas) Carbo veg 30 for 7 days

Whiteheads, rose colour, pale skin and chilly feeling Silicea 30 for 7 days

During menses, blackheads are more and worse eating sugar, fats, meat, heavy meals, tea and coffee etc. Psorinum 200 weekly one dose, total 3 doses

Blackheads are worse in summer. Use Antim crudum 30, three times a day for 7 days.

Note: If the black heads do not recede within a week, better consult a homoeopath.

Cautions for Black/Whiteheads

- Do not use cleansers having cream base, cold cream, sunscreen lotions etc. in the treatment of blackheads.
- Do not use any kind of medicated soap, cream, cosmetics or lotion without the guidance of a dermatologist. Please check the expiry date of the cream before use. An expired chemical ointment or cream may damage the face.
- Drink enough quantity of water; take fruits and green vegetables with nutritional food. Such a routine detoxifies the body.
- If you have eruptions like acne or boils on the back and chest with blackheads on the face, try to wear cotton clothes and avoid completely the use of polyesters or silky garments. Change your clothes everyday without fail.
- Do not pick or scratch the black or white heads with your nails or fingers. The eruption may aggravate.

BLEMISHES

Blemishes are called pigmentations also. Blemishes are generally considered as a precursor of pregnancy and it continues on the face even after delivery of child. Actually it is not connected with pregnancy but it shows the deficient blood and anaemic conditions. Diabetes, profuse blood flow during menses, and bleeding piles are also the causes of blemishes. It is very essential that the treatment of blemishes should be done quickly otherwise the marks of pigmentation can rarely be eliminated. Homoeopathic treatment is very beneficial and can be tried through a senior homoeopath.

The following maybe be done:

- Get your blood tested and if your haemoglobin is less. Take quality nutritional food under the advice of a doctor.
- Check your cosmetics and if you are constantly using a particular product, discontinue the same and find if any changes have come in your marks on the face. Some cosmetics give rise to blemishes.
- Avoid going into the sun during summer.
- Do not bleach your face.

Home Remedies

Take lime juice, honey and hydrogen peroxide, one teaspoon each and mix them. Apply the same on your blemishes and wash the mixture after half an hour. Continue this for at least seven days and find the difference. If you are not finding any difference try the following.

Take one almond piece and dip it in water for a night. Grind it in the morning and peel its cover off. Mix this paste in one teaspoon each of limejuice and honey and apply this paste on your face. Wash the face after half an hour. Continue this application for seven days.

Homoeopathic Medicines

The treatment should be under the guidance of a homoeopath. The medicines for treating blemishes are Berberis aqui, Cimicifuga and Sars, Sars is particularly good for young women.

CHLOASMA

During childhood or youth, if these spots are noticed, the term used for such spots is 'Chloasma' or Moth patches. It is a disorder of pigmentation. Chloasma is yellow, brown or black pigmentation of the skin and it is either multiple or single in shape. It is circumscribed or diffused.

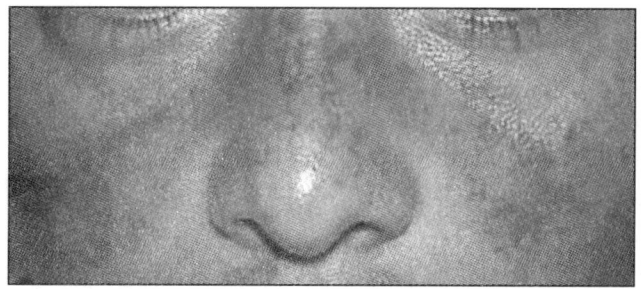

Face with chloasma

The face is commonly the target of chloasma but it can be on the chest, back, neck. If these appear on the skin, it should be differentiated from leucoderma or white patches. If it is bright white and not dusty white, it has some connection with leucoderma or white patches. It maybe due to external causes like local use of irritants, long continued friction or pressure on particular spots of the skin, and heat of cold in prolonged duration and their effects. The primary internal causes are diseases of spleen, liver, ovaries, and uterus. The brown spots seen generally on children maybe due to presence of worms in the stomach.

Homoeopathic Treatment of Chloasma

The treatment of chloasma should be under guidance of a doctor. There maybe some endocrine disorder, anaemia, gastrointestinal infestations or liver disorders and all this require treatment. As I said in the case of liver spots, I have seen good results in the use of homoeopathic Beriberi Aqua ointment (external use). Internally there are many medicines to be given and these should be under the guidance of doctor. The case generally starts with a few doses of Cina 200 and later either of Ars., Lyco, Nux-v, or sulph is selected.

DARK CIRCLES

Eyes have a vital importance in the attribution of a beautiful face. It is the eyes that expresses a person's mind. Wide eyes, black eyes, black eyebrows, and decorated eyes are of no importance if there are dark circles around the eyes. Dark circles around or beneath the eyes denote many disorders. This darkness maybe due to lack of sleep, hereditary influence or after some disease of the body.

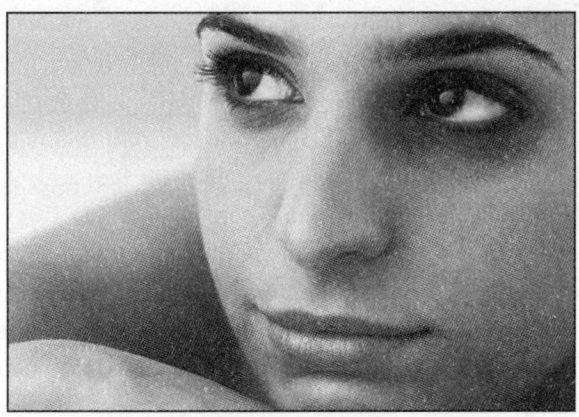

Dark circles

The skin around the eyes is very tender and soft. When this soft skin is rubbed vigorously with towel after facials or washing of the face with soaps, the skin develops minute lines after continuous rubbing for months. This skin is also rubbed more to clean the colour of the eye make-up that are used. It can be the liner or the eye-shadows. It maybe noted that the skin below the eyes has no oil glands. The result is that skin gets black or wrinkled sooner for want of proper moisture and become dry.

Treatment

- Emphasis should be on good nutritional food with lot of green vegetables, milk and yogurts. Non-vegetarian food should be avoided.
- Take enough of sleep and avoid worries/tensions.
- Externally, some treatment can be given but it helps lesser than the internal treatment as said above.
- Daily massage around the eyes can be very useful.
- Use goggles on the eyes during the day when the sun is shining brightly.
- Clean the dark circles with wet cotton pieces. Cut potatoes in very small pieces and wrap them in a very thin porous cloth. Put this cloth on the dark circles with gentle pressure. Continue this procedure for 15 minutes for 10-15 days. Find the difference.
- In summers, you may use ice cubes for compression on the dark circles for 15 minutes and see the difference after 15 days.
- Apply almond-oil over the dark circles area while going to bed and give a gentle massage for 10 minutes. Remove the oil with wet cotton pieces and go to sleep.

Homoeopathic Treatment

The medicines used for dark circles around or beneath the eyes are Ars., Carb-v, Chin, Ign, Phos-ac, Phos, Rhus-t, Sec, Stann, Staph, and Sulphur. The medicines are to be taken under the guidance of a senior homoeopath.

FRECKLES

Freckles on the face are a disease of the skin concerning pigmentation. It is most probably due to an autosomal dominant gene in the body. It starts early in the life as light brown macules on the face and mostly on the exposed parts of the body. The other parts that are exposed to the sun are neck, dorsa of hands and forearms. If sun exposure is continued on the face, the freckles go on darkening. The onset of freckles is without any other symptoms of any disease on the body. Freckles should not be confused with

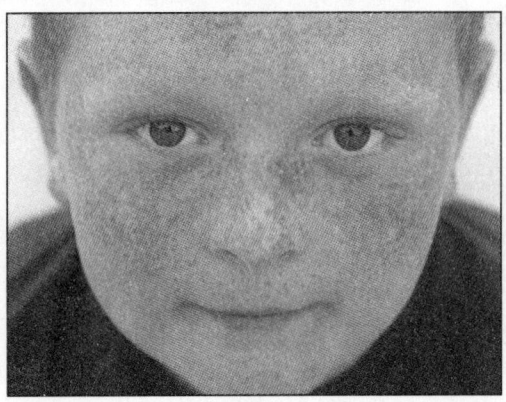

Freckles

blemishes that we have already discussed above. The skin should be protected from sunlight exposures and sunscreen creams available in the market to be used.

Treatment with Homoeopathy

The treatment should be started under the guidance of a Homoeopath. The medicines useful for removing freckles are Calcarea, Lyco, Ant-c., Phos., Puls, and sulphur.

LIVER SPOTS OR BROWN SPOTS

Many patients above the age of fifty come to doctors having brown spots on the back of their hands or arms. There is nothing that can be done for these spots as they indicate the advent of old age. There are many preparations recommended for local applications. I have given homoeopathic Beriberi aqua ointment for local application and good results are seen when used for longer periods. They become light but do not vanish. Generally, vitamin E and vitamin C is recommended by doctors to clear the spots. But the results are not encouraging.

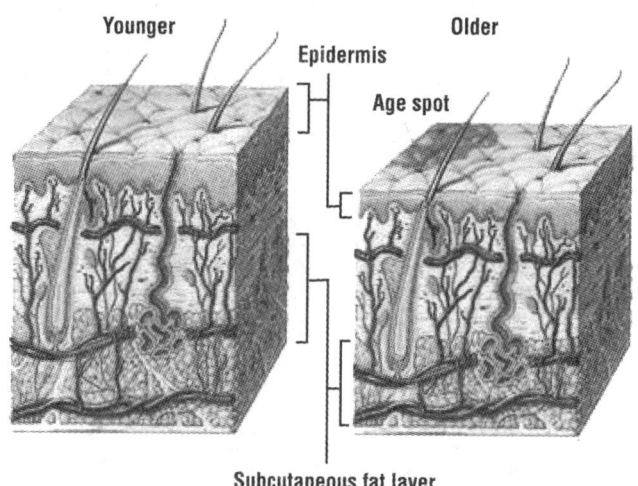

Liver spots or Brown spots

Homoeopathy

The treatment should be under the guidance of a homoeopath. The main medicines for white or circumscribed spots are Chin, Lyco, Sulph, Sepia and intermediate medicine is Tub.

MOLES/NAEVI

Under the common name of pigmentation or blemishes come the name of Moles. People do not bother about them if they are under the garments but when they are on the face or neck in clusters or groups, they appear awkward. Mole is an overabundance of pigment in the skin. When it enlarges or forms a sore, it should be got examined by a dermatologist. Sometimes, it becomes melanotic sarcoma (cancer).

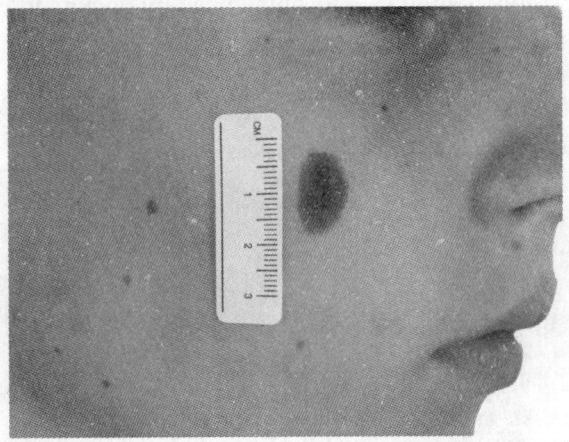
Moles/naevi

Common variety of moles is absolutely harmless. They maybe large, raised a little above the skin, black, brown, or hairy. One should watch them in the beginning for they may get bigger. If they remain the same size for years, there is no danger. Most of the moles in flat-pigmented form are harmless and even taken as identity marks when making biodata in service records of officers. Moles are also considered as beauty spots.

Treatment

If the person does not like the harmless moles, they can be got removed easily from the cosmetic surgeon. The removal of spots do not leave scars. The following scrub can be used for very little moles that have recently erupted and not by birth.

Take barley flour, remains of wheat flour and sieve them. When flour is filtered, add rice flour and grinded almonds each in one-teaspoon quantity.

Almond powder is to be made out of ten pieces. Mix them all in water to make a paste. Apply the scrub on the face and rub the face to and fro with strokes with your hands. Wash the face thoroughly with fresh water.

Homoeopathy

Calcarea, Carbo-v, Graphite, Nit-ac, Petr, Ph-ac, Puls, Sil, Sul-ac, Sulph, Terent, and thujare the medicines useful to remove the moles. It takes long time to remove the moles but I have seen good results. At least the future eruption of moles is immediately stopped once the treatment starts. The medicines should be taken under the guidance of a homoeopath.

WRINKLES OF FACE

Wrinkles are folds on the skin which is supposed to be smooth. If they appear before the ageing of the skin, which is in the old age, the wrinkles can be handled or got faded by means of massage, and some beauty products. It is the facial wrinkles that disturb the women. The massage of the face has to be done in such a manner that it does not hurt the skin or create scratches. 'Of all the methods of beautifying the skin, one of which is considered fundamental is contraction', says Dr S. Siddantalankar in his book 'From Old age to youth through Yoga'. Why does the formation of folds start hanging beneath the neck? Why does skin become loose? All this happens because the skin loses its capacity for contraction and relaxation which means that it loses its elasticity.

Premature wrinkles of the face are due to UV rays of the sun and it is said that UV rays account for 80 percent of the cases of premature wrinkles. These rays not only affect the outer surface of the skin but also go deep into the skin and remove the moisture to make it dry. Dryness in turn brings in rashes, itching and wrinkles The kin develops folds that start hanging. To remove the wrinkles of the face, one should not try any kind of massage on the face by herself or himself but prefer to take advice from a beauty expert. Facial massages done at the beauty parlours are beneficial provided they are under the guidance of some famous beautician. The massages at home are not recommended and what can be done at home is the application of beauty masks.

Use of Scrubs for Wrinkles

The process of scrub is to rub hard with something coarse. There are many scrubs available in the market but it is wise to prepare a scrub at home. A few recipes are given below for the readers.

Scrub number-1

Take barley flour, remains of wheat flour and sieve them. When the flour is filtered, add rice flour and grinded almonds each in one-teaspoon quantity.

Almond powder is to be made out of ten pieces. Mix them all in water to make a paste. Apply the scrub on the face with strokes of your hands and rub on the face to and fro. Wash the face thoroughly with fresh water.

Scrub number 2

Remove skins of oranges and lemons. Grind them separately to make a teaspoon of powder. Mix them together. Add one teaspoon of barley flour. Add one teaspoon of powdered almonds. Add one spoonful of rose water and make a paste.

Scrub the paste on the face for some time and then wash the face. This can be done once a week to remove the wrinkles and if the skin is oily, do it thrice a week.

Rules for Application of Masks

Mask application is an art. You have to prepare your face before wearing a mask. First of all, tie your so that the hair does not come on the face. Next step is either use some cleanser or a scrub. After this, apply the mask on the face with the help of some wide and soft brush. Do not apply mask on the eyelids, the area around the eyes and lips. Mask should be left for fifteen minutes to dry before washing.

Mask of Vegetables and Fruits

Carrot and cabbage mask is very good for wrinkle removal. All the items are to be boiled first. Filter the vegetables so that water is separated. Let the water and vegetable mash cool down. Wash the face with the filtered water. Now apply the remains of the vegetables or the mash as mask on the face and let it remain there for 15 minutes. In the same manner mask of fruits can be used with banana, apple and papaya.

Mask of Cornflakes

Take three tablespoon of cornflakes. Mix one teaspoon of milk, honey and white of egg. Make a paste and apply on the face. Let it remain for fifteen minutes and then wash the face.

Mask of Egg White

Those who have no objection to the use of eggs should apply the white portion of an egg on the wrinkles and leave it for 4-5 minutes before wiping it out. The contracting effect of the egg white will remove the wrinkles and the skin will look smooth. Such a strong astringent should not be allowed to remain on the wrinkles for more than 4-5 minutes otherwise it may cause the skin to shrink thus deepening the wrinkles.

Non-vegetarian Toner Mask

Take one tablespoon of yogurt and one tablespoon of fuller's earth. Mix them.

Take the white portion of one egg. Add this white of egg and mix thoroughly with yogurt and fuller's earth. Apply this on your face and let it dry. After it is dry, rinse it off with water. Do not let it remain on your face after the mixture gets dry. The mask can be applied every fourth day.

Cleansing Mask Fuller's Earth

Take one-fourth cup of fuller's earth and add some pulp of tomato. Keep this mixture aside.

Take two tablespoonful of yogurt and one teaspoonful of cucumber juice. Mix them thoroughly. Mix both the first and second mixtures together and again stir them to make a paste. The mask is ready. Apply this mask on your face and wait for fifteen to twenty minutes. Rinse the mask away with moderate cold water. Every third day this should be done to diminish the wrinkles.

Other Means for Removal of Wrinkles of Face

Some beauty experts say that the use of Aloe-Vera gel (available in the market) on the wrinkles is beneficial. Grinded coriander paste is good for wrinkles removal. Massage of coconut oil on the wrinkles before going to sleep is good. Taking honey with pieces of ginger in the morning is very good for wrinkles-removal. Pack of honey and gram flour when applied on the face fades away wrinkles.

Homoeopathic Treatment of Wrinkles

The premature wrinkles of the face due to any reason can be treated in Homoeopathy. The main medicines are Abort, Alum, Calc, Lyco, and Syph. They should be taken under the guidance of a senior doctor.

WARTS

Warts are viral infections on the skin and they look like small or big eruptions in white, pink or brown/black colour. These eruptions grows only on the epidermis or outer portion of the skin. They are slightly raised, hanging or flat-topped. We shall not go into the details of how they occur but seek treatment. If you happen to get warts and have shown to a dermatologist, the advice would have been surgical removal of warts. Allopathic system of medicine does not have its internal treatment.

If the warts are not treated in time, the infection multiplies and more of warts come up being a viral infection. If they are not multiplying they are not warts but skin-tags. Skin tags have to be removed surgically and homoeopathy has no medicine for them. Common warts that occur on the face, neck, armpits, dorsum of hands and arms have to be treated by a homoeopath and you cannot help remove it with the help of any domestic tool. Thuja is a well-known medicine for warts of all types and I have seen people self-prescribing this medicine. Do not practice this. It can be dangerous and you can have more of warts instead of cure.

Homoeopathy

Antim crud., Calcarea, Natrum sulf, Dulca, Ars., Sabina, Nat-mur and many other medicines are useful for removal of warts. Contact a senior Homoeopath of your locality.

Chapter 12

Hirsutism

UNWANTED HAIR GROWTH ON THE FACE

A smooth, clean, shining face without any hair growth on the face is a desire that have always haunted the ladies. Hair on the other parts of the body can be adjusted by hiding the same but hiding the face becomes nearly impossible. Most of the times such a hair growth is not very prominent but ladies are very conscious about it. Growth of hair at abnormal sites of the body is a condition called hypertrichosis.

It is usually confined to those cases in which a growth of thick hair occurs in the sites usually covered with lanugos hairs, such as the face in women. Most of the ladies maintain a hidden depression about the growth of hair on unwanted sites of the body. Women sometimes develop a sort of inferiority complex whenever there is a gathering or social function and there is possibility of beauty being discussed in the functions. They are hesitant to shave the facial hairs as there is myth that hair grows more speedily increases when they are shaved. We shall discuss about the solution to this problem as this is a vital contributory factor which adds to the beauty of one's face.

Dermal tumours and sites of melanocytic nevi also have this growth of hair on them. Sometimes thick hair are present on pigmented moles and they are seldom larger than several square centimeters. In women, excessive hair growth on unwanted sites is known as 'Hirsutism' although hypertrichosis is considered to be a more right word. The disorder varies from a few strong hairs on each side of the chin to profuse growth affecting the area near the upper lips, cheeks, chin, and the neck. In some cases, the growth is also on the centre of the breasts, the lower abdomen, and the groins. The growth of hair on the face is sometimes so much that people call the woman as 'bearded'.

Indian women have little hirsutism if they are compared with the women of other countries. Many races of Russian, South European, and Middle East women have hirsutism more than their Indian counterparts.

CAUSES

In many cases, hirsutism is congenital. If the pregnant woman takes excessive drugs, the baby born might have hirsutism with features like wide, large lips and mouth and a short neck. Congenital syphilis is also one of the reasons for this disease. The hair is often shed extensively but on the other hand, syphilitic infants may grow an abundant crop of hair, which has been called the 'syphilitic mop' though it occurs in other diseases.

In cases where hirsutism is acquired, it may be a result of lipoatrophic diabetes and other syndromes like, Lange, Hurler, and Morogu etc. Use of some typical steroids also becomes cause of hypertrichosis. Use of androgens and certain high progesterone birth control pills (though not so common) also cause hirsutism. Use of drugs like costicosteroids, phenytoin, diazoxide and minoxidil are also reported to produce hirsutism.

It is not necessary that these drugs will produce hairs on the face only. These can produce abundance of hair-growth on any part of the body. In cases where limbs have grown more than the rest of body (disproportionate- a condition called 'Acromegaly'), the growth of hair is more. Hormonal changes in the body also make a difference. Hirsutism maybe due to excessive secretion of androgens from either ovary of adrenal gland or from excessive stimulation by pituitary tumours. The secretions in excess maybe due to functional excesses or from neoplastic processes.

Hirsutism can develop at any age but it is observed that women reaching menopause develop more of it on their faces. It is possibly some endocrine disorder as well. Another cause is said to be extra precautions that ladies take when they grow old. They use vaseline, cold creams and greasy applications repeatedly to cover wrinkles. Such greasy cosmetics may cause excessive hair growth. It is also seen in some cases that hirsutism is associated with signs of virilization that has balding at temples, deepening of voice, acne and clitoral hypertrophy.

PROGNOSIS

The prognosis is both good and bad. Good, because the hair can be removed mechanically and cosmetic methods now available in the market and there is nothing to worry about. It is bad, because there is no permanent solution to remove hair by the intake of internal medicines.

You will find very occasionally a male seeking advice regarding hirsutism on the trunk, a condition that is seen in a proportion of males.

This condition does not constitute an abnormality. It is also seen that strong hair are found on pigmented moles and these moles are large in some cases. But still these people are not bothered about them because these are seldom larger than a few square centimeters. Also, a tuft of well-developed long hair is seen arising from the skin overlying a spina bifida (a congenital defect in which the vertebral neural arches fail to close) in some cases but males do not bother about these as well.

TREATMENT

Women have been very much conscious about their looks from times immemorial. There are many methods available for removal of hair. Both cosmetics and mechanical methods exist but shaving is the best method though it is not liked due to social restrictions. Some women use a piece of soaped pumice stone to scrub away the hair instead of using a razor. There are waxes (epilatory) and chemical depilatories available in the market which women use. (Both the terms depilatory and epilatory mean removal of hair. The constituents in both make them different)

Hair Removing Creams and Wax

The depilatory remedies are not injurious and they are not so costly. Every brand of hair removing cream or wax or soap available in the market has its secret formula. In all these preparations, the sulphides of barium and calcium are commonly used. Sulphide of barium is mixed with equal parts of oxide of zinc and starch to make a thick cream with water. This cream is spread on the hairs to be removed and allowed to dry for ten minutes after which it is washed. Most of the products carry instructions with them for the removal procedure. Most of women prefer epilating waxes. Epilating waxes are made of beeswax and rosin. Wax removes the hairs temporarily. Epilatory waxes have advantages over depilatory waxes because their use is not attended with the risk of inflammation, eczema or chemical burns.

However, a patch test is needed before the use of epilating

waxes/hair remover cream. The other method of removing hairs is bleaching. Bleaching the hair with equal parts of hydrogen peroxide and liquid ammonia makes them less conspicuous and has a beneficial corrosive action on the finer hair. It makes the hair less dark and thus less noticeable. Bleaching should not be done at home and preferably should be done from beauty parlours.

Some women resort to endocrine therapy (hormonal) including use of the newer ovarian preparations. This method is mostly disappointing. There is a notion that removal of hair by plucking, shaving or waxing brings more of hair growth in the area. This has been proved false.

REMOVAL OF HAIR

Hair Removal by Electrolysis

One of the oldest method is 'Electrolysis'. Electrolysis consists in passing a current of about 1 miliampere for quarter to half a minute into the hair bulb by means of a fine needle attached to the negative pole of a galvanic battery. The hair thus loosens and can be removed. It is very essential that the hair be not removed too close to one another at the same sitting. If it is done in one sitting, there maybe troublesome scar left. The experts working in beauty parlours take care of it. A still modified method of electrolysis is pulsed light treatment that takes about five to six sittings for removal of hair. This is painless and there are no marks left on the skin.

Other Methods

'Diathermy coagulation' is another mode that is considered satisfactory treatment of hypertrichosis of moderate degree on the face and also for removal of hair from the moles. With the advent of science, the beauty experts have now introduced permanent 'excess body hair removal method' called 'Light sheer diode laser' method. This method claims that no further growth of hair will take place. In electrolysis and diathermy coagulation, therepetition of removal of hair is needed after some period. I am not very sure about this term 'permanent removal' in light sheer diode laser method and it sounds like 'permanent' hair-dyes that do not colour the hair permanently. My knowledge about the advantages and disadvantages of this method is limited since this is a new invention. Before going in for this method, one should get hold of the complete details about the re-growth of hair. Nevertheless, new claims are supposed to be better than the old ones.

Domestic Preparations for Temporary Hair Removal

1. Grind about two tablespoons of gram and make a powder. Mix same quantity of fenugreek powder. Make a thick paste with some water and apply on the area from where you want to remove hair. After this is dried on the skin, rub it clean making a movement in the opposite direction of the hair. You will find that after applying this for a few times, the hair is completely removed. There will be no growth for some weeks and after you feel that the growth is occurring again, repeat the procedure.

2. In a vessel, take one cup of water and one cup of sugar. Heat the mixture till the mixture is thick. Remove the vessel from heat and when the mixture is slightly warm, apply it on the desired area. Rub mildly in the opposite direction of their growth. The hair will be removed and will grow after many weeks and the same mixture can be used again.

3. Take 500 gms of water and mix in it 1 cup of sugar. Heat this mixture till the sugar gets dissolved in the water. Take one-fourth teaspoon of citric acid and half teaspoon of glycerin

dissolved in half cup of warm water. Now add this mixture in sugar water already made. Mix them thoroughly and use it to remove hair.
4. Take thick granules of sugar, add lemon juice in it and then rub the sugar to the hairy parts of your legs and arms. Better not to try this on face because the scrubbing of sugar on the face, being very soft, may bring rashes.

How is Waxing Done?

Instead of making wax at home, if you opt to use the hair removal waxes available in the market, it will be better. You will get the manual with the wax telling you how it should be applied and how to remove and hair from the face, legs, arms, underarms etc. You will require to do this removing of hair every month nearly.

At first, wash the area from where the hair is to be removed and dry it with soft towel. The hair removing wax is to be applied in the direction of the hair growth with the applicator supplied with the cream. Wait for some time as prescribed in the directions of the usage of the wax. Now put a piece of cloth in the opposite direction of growth of the hair. The cloth is then pulled in the opposite direction pulling out the hair from their follicles. Take 5 pills of Rhus tox 30, a homoeopathic medicine before application and then after application, take 5 pills of Arnica 30 in case you have some skin allergy and there is an eruption of small bumps on the skin. Alternatively, one tablet of Avil can be taken after the allergy appears.

How is Shaving Done?

This is the easiest method to remove the hair. Shaving is preferred on all parts of the body except face where the shaved area looks awkward after the hair growth takes place. If shaving is started it has to be done on weekly basis. A good quality razor is to be used for the shaving so that no cuts occur. Apply some moisturizer or even coconut oil before using a razor and after a minute wash the area. Soak it dry with a soft towel. Now apply shaving cream wetting the brush and lather it up.

On legs and arms or armpits, use the razor in long strokes from down to up.

Tweezing Method

For removing gray hair people use this method of tweezing. For removing of hair growth on the face or the eye brows, this method is not recommended. Pulling hair from the roots is painful and sometimes it leaves scars or pitting of skin.

Treatment in Homoeopathy

Many experts claim that they have cured cases of hirsutism but my practical experience is different. People come for treatment but leave the medicines before they even start acting. The time taken is long and the people have no patience. I am talking of acquired hirsutism. Congenital hirsutism has less chances of cure. Following opinions maybe considered to start an effective treatment.

Dr R.B. Bishambar Das, author of 'Select your Remedy' suggests that Oleum Jec may be given in 30 potency in summer and in 3x potency in winter thrice daily along with Thuja 1M. Oleum is not to be given two days before or after giving Thuja.

Besides this, he suggests that a mechanical method should be adopted for the removal of facial hair. He advises that yellow sulphate of arsenic and quick lime in equal parts be mixed in hot water to make a paste. This paste should be applied on the face and allowed to dry. No hair will show there for weeks.

Dr J.N.Shinghal suggests that Thuja 200 should be given every month and Oleum-jec 3x be given thrice daily except on the day when Thuja is taken. Dr T.P. Chatterjee says that Thuja 200 should be given weekly and Oleum-jec 3x be given twice daily excepting the day on which Thuja is taken till the growth stops. Further for growth of excessive hair on a child's face, Calc, Nat-m, Ol-j, Psor and Sulph should be tried according to the symptoms of the body. Actually, Kent suggests the same for a child's facial hair growth.

According to Kent's repertory for hair on unusual parts, there are two medicines indicated, Med and Thuj. The same is for treatment of Hairy parts.

Note: It is better not to try these prescriptions. These views of doctors are given to benefit other doctors. Better consult a doctor for homoeopathic treatment.

Do not Hesitate

One thing is sure that by removal of unwanted hair from the face, the person gets mental satisfaction. Women visit beauty parlours frequently for jobs like threading, bleaching, facial, manicure, pedicure, massages and haircuts. Why to hesitate for facial hair removal? It infuses confidence when you are standing before the mirror. Do not let your mind remain sorrowful on this account. Forget that it is a disorder. Include it in your routine of beauty-culture.

Chapter 13

Yoga and Beauty

Today, both male and especially female throng in beauty parlours for maintaining external beauty. But there is an entity called internal beauty. This internal beauty when taken care of will help to enhance the external beauty also through the system of Yoga.

WHAT IS YOGA?

If someone has studied the therapy of Chinese Acupuncture, he or she must be knowing that there are about seven hundred points in the body which when punctured relieves the body of ailments. Chinese believe it to be oldest the traditional therapy. What about our Indian Yoga? Lately, people of India have developed a deep belief that yoga can make one healthy in a better way than acupuncture.

Yoga has proved to be great healer of diseases as has been

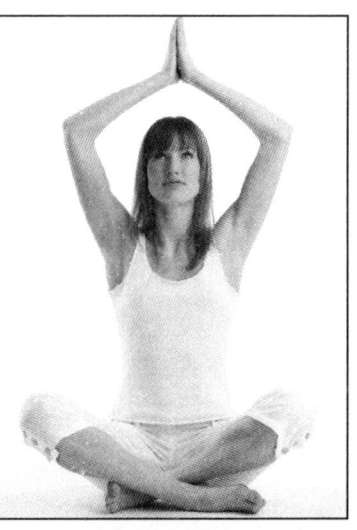

The art of yoga

demonstrated by Swami Ramdev of Haridwar in India. Credit for the spread of Yoga goes to this great man.

In Yoga, there are only seven, not seven hundred energy points if we compare acupuncture with yoga. These are called seven 'Chakra' of the body. Each Chakra may have one hundred points or so. For instance, there is a 'sexual' sphere in the body and it has one hundred energy points scattered on different parts of the body. These points are called erotic zones of the body. By touching these erotic zones by the opposite sex, the energy flows from them and one gets the expected pleasure-results during intercourse.

According to latest research, the lower lobes of ears have tremendous energy points or erotic points. These points are very sensitive. You must have seen many Indian saints and even old persons with holes in their ear lobes. If you closely see the photo or statue of the renowned saints of different cults as displayed in many temples, you will find their ears lobes unusually long and having holes. See the statues of Lord Mahabir and Lord Buddha. You will be surprised that their ears appear to be touching their shoulders and having holes as well. I have lived in jungles and remote mountains where I came across many such saints who have made a big hole in the ear lobes and they were wearing a type of earring made of elephant teeth.

The purpose of such holes, as told by these saints, is their absolute intention to control their sexual urges. By doing so, their so-called sexual energy is converted into spiritual energy and absorbed in their body-Chakra. Such conserved energy could thus be utilized for the benefit of the mankind. When I enquired from them about the source of this information, they explained that it was from the ancient 'Yoga' system that they had gained this knowledge which in turn was given in ancient religious books. Smearing the forehead with ash or sandal or even drawing various types of 'Tilak' on the forehead has also the same reason of strengthening the chakras of the body. The central point between two eyebrows is the point of wisdom-energy, which is awakened and triggered by the application of coolants like ash, sandal powder and vermilion.

The set of exercises called 'yogasanas' are supposed to trigger certain body points where our 'energy' is centred. By exerting pressure on certain vital points of the body by means of yogasanas, we attract and pull energy of the body from other strong points of the body to that particular weak organ to activate it. The energy from other points is drawn to the pressure point and the part targeted for cure gets vitalized or healed through better circulation of blood.

There remains no doubt that yoga has surprising effect on the body because we touch the vital energy points of the body. In the same manner, when the breathing exercise called 'Pranayam' is conducted in Yoga, it triggers the strength of lungs, cleans the blood, and adds beauty to the body.

Art of proper breathing is called 'Pranayam'. A correct and balanced method of breathing of oxygen is helpful in fighting all types of diseases of the body including the skin and the body feels relaxed although breathing is an involuntary process. It is better to watch your breathing once in a while during the daytime and correct it if it is too slow, too long and exerting you to breathe. During the sleep, if the nose is blocked, it is not good for health. If you breathe through mouth, you are allowing only dry air to enter your lungs. Dry air can lead to bronchitis.

When you breathe through nose, the dry air is mixed with humidity in the nasal air passage and is filtered as well. This prevents sinusitis. If the breathing is not proper, there would be lack of oxygen in the body. 'Proper breathing' means that breathing should be such that you do not feel any exertion while taking in the oxygen. It should not be too deep and too often because this would mean losing too much carbon dioxide. Losing too much carbondioxide can upset the acid/alkaline balance in the body. Similarly, breathing out too often could trigger inefficient metabolism. Too deep, too often breathing in and too deep, too often breathing out is called improper breathing. Please take note that the above statement is not for those who might conduct the above method during pranayam because pranayam is an exercise. Not only that, the oxygen level in the body should be accurate; but also the level of carbon dioxide should be normal. If the level of carbon dioxide in the blood is less than normal, excessive oxygen could cause joint and muscles pain.

In Australia, the scientists have developed a breathing technique called 'Buteyko' and people are being trained for breathing correctly so that they are not deficient of carbon dioxide. (Courtesy: Times news network—'Times life' dated March 5, 2006) Some people suffer from obstructive sleep apnea (OSA), which is due to shallow breathing. Shallow breathing can lead to heart and lungs disorders and hypertension. The best way to avoid OSA is to get checked for nasal polyps or fat deposits in the nasal passage. As soon as one feels more of sleepiness during the daytime and easy fatigue, it is time to get the nose checked. At home, intake of breaths with steam helps and of course the best is pranayam.

PRANAYAM, THE CORRECT BREATHING

In Yoga, we have a method of correct breathing. A person conducting Yoga has to breathe in deeply with every asana and leave the breathing slowly at certain junctures of asanas. Without this breathing technique, yoga is incomplete. The proper technique of breathing in and out is called pranayam.

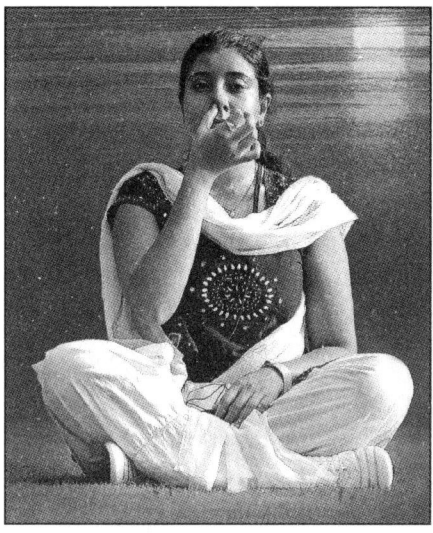

Pranayam, the correct way of breathing

Pranayam is not merely a breathing technique by which the respiratory system is rectified but an effective method to improve the circulation of blood and purify the blood with the help of air we breathe in. You have observed that complexion of majority of people living in the hills are fair and healthy. The race and heredity plays a part in this but the fresh air they breathe in plays a major part. Breathing in and out is also associated with walking up and down the hills. Both fresh air and the exertion of walking makes a positive effect on the skin.

In the plains, we do not have fresh air. To make our complexion good and fair, we have to follow the pattern of hilly people. Pranayam can substitute hill's fresh air provided it is done in the morning when air in the city-parks is not polluted.

Curing Diseases by Pranayam

Pranayam helps the lungs to purify the blood through deep

and systematic breathing of air. The process of breathing in and breathing out impart life giving oxygen to our blood and eliminate carbon dioxide. We generally breathe impure air and hence get easily fatigues due to more accumulation of carbon dioxide. This is the reason when we go to some hill resorts, we feel very fresh because there is pure air in the hills. In the planes, we need abundance of pure oxygen and that can be collected early in the morning in city gardens and also by the help of Pranayam. Pranayam aids the process of contraction and relaxation. When we inhale and retain the air in the lungs, they expand and exert pressure on the diaphragm. The pressure of diaphragm in turn puts pressure on abdominal organs. Whole of this process is called contraction and when we release the air from lungs, this spell is termed as relaxation. Contraction and relaxation actually activates the circulation of blood in the body.

When the blood circulation comes to its 'activated level', its pace removes all sorts of debris and foreign matters from the arteries and veins enabling the body a free flow of blood to all the parts of the body. The skin gets renovated and one feels very fresh and in high spirits. All the diseases of the skin vanish in a couple of months when Pranayam is done regularly.

How to Conduct Pranayam?

The initial manifestation of life in a newborn baby is to take a deep breath. This first breathing is called 'prana' meaning life because without it the baby will not survive. This ritual is without any training to the baby who takes breathing inside, retains it for a while, and then releases the breathing. This is the process of breathing against which life commences. The life ends when this breathing ceases to exist. One can live without food or water for sometime but one cannot live without breathing. To attain good health, breathing has to be controlled and vitalized by some method of *breathing in* and *breathing out*. Pranayama is developed to look into this very aspect.

Our ancient books on health reveal that there are three steps in conducting Pranayama. Inhaling air into the lungs with all one's strength is the first step called 'Poorak'. Holding back the air in the lungs is the second step called 'Kumbhak'. Final exhaling the air from the lungs is the third step called 'Rechak'. Poorak should be for about 10 seconds, Kumbhak should be for about 40 seconds and Rechak should be for 20 seconds. Actually, this depends upon the capacity of the individual and is variable.

Pranayama is the process of breathing smoothly, inhaling and exhaling from the nostrils as per following procedure:

1. Take long breaths slowly and exhale in the same way slowly. Repeat this for five minutes. This is called 'Bharstika' pranayam.
2. Inhale through the right nostril and exhale through the left nostril, using your thumb and middle finger to close and open alternate nostril by pressing side of the nose. Do it for at least for ten minutes. This is 'Anulome-Vilom' pranayam.
3. Now comes the next step. Inhale through the left nostril and hold your breath for some seconds. Now release the breath from the right nostril. For inhaling and exhaling from different side nostrils, you have to use thumb and finger to close the nostril. Do not go beyond your capacity of holding the breath. This requires practice. The time you can hold should be your capacity to do so. And in no case any longer time should be given beyond your capacity. This exercise creates a cooling effect in the body and increases the immunity. Do it for three times only.
4. Release the breathing out with a slight force so that your abdomen goes inside with the intake of air and comes back

in the same position when taking another breath-in. This means you have to do Rechak only. This is called 'Kapalbhati' pranayam. Do this pranayam for five minutes. You can start for one minute and raise it slowly up to five minutes slowly after few days.

YOGA AND SKIN

Yoga is a set of exercises and postures to make movement in the body. It is a great phenomenon of life aimed to achieve a state of mental, physical, and spiritual alignment or attainment through practice of various postures making in the body. Yoga in Sanskrit means union and it is indeed a union between the mental, physical and spiritual training.

In Yoga, the postures made of the body are called 'Asanas'. Yoga is the most honorable and pious heritage of Indian culture practiced since ages. Asanas were developed thousands of years back. Naturally, time has made them perfect. They are therefore time tested for their benefits both on internal and external body. The Yogasanas allow the body to relax and increase the flexibility of the body that brings overall fitness. They are done with a slow, stretching, and releasing of body muscles and they certainly look graceful.

Yogasanas for Healthy Skin

There are tens asanas and every one has its own benefit depending upon the body part under a pose. If the stomach is involved that is, bending the stomach muscles on folded legs (sitting on folded legs and knees backwards), there is natural benefit to the stomach muscles. In the same way the asanas are trimmed and tailored to fit all the parts of body. I have selected only two asanas for the beauty of the skin and removal of the minor skin diseases. Although, one more could be added to the list but that involves training. It is difficult also although very common. It is 'Surya-Namaskar'. If you know it, do it regularly and there is no other asana to be done for upkeep of the skin. Those who have not much of time to even learn about this 'Surya Namaskar', better the follow routined asanas.

SARVANGASAN (STANDING ON SHOULDERS)

It influences the whole body and its functions, activates the circulation of the body and brings freshness to the texture of skin, particularly the facial complexion to its original colour. Lie down on the floor and then raise both your legs towards the sky. Give a support to your loins and back by placing hands behind you. The position should be that your hands should be pressed on your back, your elbows/forearms will rest on the floor, and the legs should be towards the sky. The trunk and the neck should make a ninety-degree angle between themselves. The chin should be touching the chest. Keep your eyes stuck to both the toes of your feet. Hold on to this posture for some time according to your capacity and bring back the legs to the ground very slowly and without any jerks. The time of this posture can be increased according to the advice of your trainer. There is always a need of a trainer to learn this art.

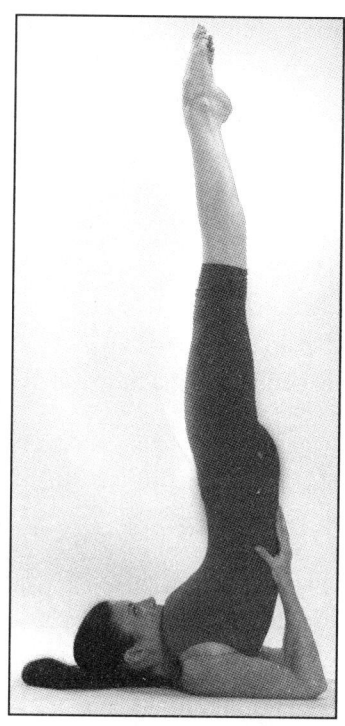

Sarvangasan

Advantages

This asana gives exercise to the neck and removes obstructions in the passage to the respiratory organs that is nostrils, olfactory area, sinuses, throat, thyroid and wind pipe thus making a complete free passage for oxygen which is very useful to remove skin disorders. Since the blood is circulated towards the face, the complexion of the face brightens.

SHAVASANA (CORPSE POSE)

After you have done Sarvangasana, keep lying flat on your back on the floor and spread your feet keeping them at a distance of about two feet. It is time for rest. Place a small pillow or folded blanket below your head. Do not use a thick pillow. Your hands should be close to your body, touching the body. The palms should face upwards and hands should not be clenched. Close your eyes. Now feel relaxed and let your body be released and let loose. Try to feel the different parts of your body in contact with the floor.

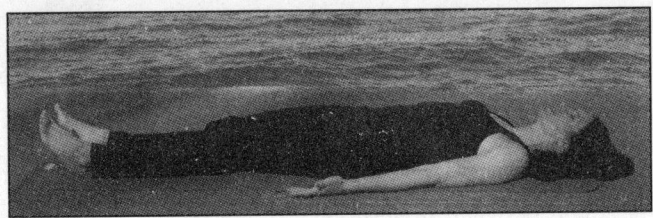

Shavasana

For doing this, close your eyes and imagine your entire body, part by part is in touch with ground and is getting heavy. Do not get worried over this when you actually feel the limbs heavy. Throughout the practice of this asana, the worries and problems may keep appearing. Convince and tell yourself that these problems will receive your attention after a few minutes and that you are now practicing shavasana.

Gently and slowly you will gain confidence and you will feel relaxed in all respects.

During the whole of asana, feel free and relaxed as if you are dead so far as your body is concerned. Remain like this at least for ten minutes without any movement. While you are acting like a corpse, breathe deeply and take long breaths.

Advantages

This asana is particularly useful for those persons who are always under tension, stress, and worries. This asana will recapture the shine of the skin and bring in lost vitality of mind.

TARH-ASANA

Stand erect and raise both your hands slowly. Along with this, raise your heels upwards. Now entangle both hands' fingers with each other when the arms are up in full length. Keep the neck straight and look upwards. Keep this pose for a while till you can stand. Lower your hands and heels back on the ground. Your breathing has to be normal during the course of this asana.

If you are unable to do this standing without any support, you can enact the whole of asana by standing against the wall and raising the heels. The heels in this case should be resting on the wall and toes should be on the floor.

Advantages

This asana will reduce the fat of your stomach and the height of the person is also increased provided he or she is below 16 years of age and has no body ailment.

KON-ASANA

Stand on the floor in the erect position and widen your legs. Keep both your hands on the waist and bend towards right. Be in this position for some time and then come back to the erect position. Now bend towards the left. Be there for some time and come back to the erect position. Do this left and right exercise for ten times daily.

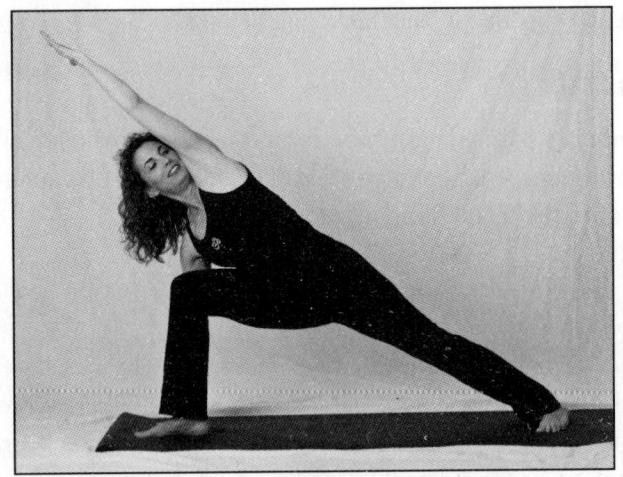

Kon-asana

Advantages

Blood circulation is corrected and it adds to your beauty. The waist gets thin and its fat is lost.

Note: Pranayam and Yogasans should not be done without proper guidance and training by a master.

BI-WEEKLY BODY MASSAGE

If you want to have a healthy skin and glowing look on your face, it is a must that you have to give massage to your body at least twice a week. If you cannot do it yourself, you can engage a person for this or go to a massage parlour.

At the age around forty, the skin of the body starts getting folds and wrinkles. We have already read that the dermis, which is the real skin, contains muscles and capillaries needs activation. Above the dermis is epidermis; it is the upper layer of the skin that you see.

It is the dermis that has to be strengthened so that no folds etc. are seen on the epidermis and the skin shines. Activating the skin through massage can only do this strengthening. This massage when transmitted to the dermis activates the blood circulation and opens the capillaries. This means there should be frictional effort on the epidermis. This friction can be made by a massage. The more is the friction, the more is the activation of the dermis. Muscles at or around forty years of age become weak and a simple massage would not do any harm. This massage has to be associated with oil so that the skin is lubricated as well.

For massaging the body, mustard oil is the best. In case you feel that it is too oily, it can be replaced by Olive oil. Mustard oil may create stickiness but olive oil is free from it. It does not spoil the clothes whereas mustard oil spoils the clothes. The massage of the body should be done from down to the upward direction starting from the legs towards the thighs. Then is the turn of buttocks and the loins. Every stroke of the oiled hand should be directed towards the heart. The massage of the abdomen and the chest can be done sideways and then the arms. Massage of the arms should start from the wrists making strokes towards the arm and the forearm. The back should be massaged by someone else. Massage of head should be done daily but the whole body massage can be done twice in a week. Massage keeps the skin young and healthy. This routine of massage should be bi-weekly for better results. A professional may be hired for correct massaging of the body.

Chapter 14

Normal Values of Weight, Height and Laboratory Findings

Knowing the normal weight of the body is a relevant subject in terms of a beautiful slim body. When I was about to complete this book and give it the finishing touches, it struck me that the book must give knowledge about the normal weight, normal height, and the laboratory findings. Not particularly in the case of beauty problems but in all spheres of life when a person in the family is suddenly ill, he or she is advised laboratory test. One should know the normal values of results of test because the laboratories official do not tell about the results and refer back to doctors. The period when you consult a doctor and the period the report is lying with the patient is stressful. This chapter of the book will help you and your relatives to find out the results for yourself. Of course, some doctor has to be consulted who advised the tests.

NORMAL WEIGHT AND HEIGHT CHART

Height (Cm)Weight (Kg)	Male	Female
148	47.5	46.5
152	49	48.5
156	51.5	50
160	53.5	52.5
164	56	55
172	62	60.5
176	65.5	64
180	68.5	67
184	72	69

1st Method

The over weight and underweight can be estimated by giving a margin of 20% to the values given above. Here is an example. If the weight is 49, the overweight will be 59 and underweight will be 39. If the weight is 55, the overweight will be 66 and the underweight will be 44. This is just a rough estimate and should not considered reliable.

2nd Method

For a general height of 5 feet, the normal weight of the body is 50 kg. For every inch beyond five feet, add 2 kg extra. If you were five feet and two inches, the normal weight should be 50 kg plus 2 inches multiplied by 2 which is equal to 4 kg. Now add 4 kg to 50 that makes 54 kg. This is an average calculation both for men and women.

3rd Method, BMI

Another method of finding out the exact weight is body mass index is given below. Body mass index can be calculated by converting your weight into kilograms. Now convert your height into metres and then make square of it. Divide weight by the height. If your weight is 65 kg and height is 1.68 metres. The Square of 1.68 is 1.68 multiplied by 1.68, which comes to 2.82. Now divide 65 by 2.82. The body mass index is 23.0.

Square of height in metres H2 Normal values in men range from 20 to 25 and in women it is 19 to 24. A BMI over 25 is distinct in obesity. A chart of normal values of BMI is available in the market.

LABORATORY FINDINGS

Blood Values Normal Value

- WBC (white blood cells) 5000-10,000/cu mm
- Neutrophils 60 to 70 %
- Eosinophils 1-4 %

Eosinophil increase is due to hyper immune, allergic and degenerative reaction, parasitic diseases, lung and bone cancer and Hodgkin's diseases. Leucocytosis up to 50,000 is high, 30,000 is moderate and 20,000 is slight. Causes of leucocytosis is infection, hemorrhage, toxins, after certain drugs, serum sickness and after steroids.

RBC (Red blood cells) 4.2 to 5.4 million/cu mm (men) 3.6 to 5 million/cu mm (women). Decreased value means anaemia, leukemia, Hodgkin disease, rheumatic fever, and infective endocarditis. Increased values mean polycythemia vera, severe diarrhea, dehydration and acute poisoning.

ESR Men- 0-15 mm per hour; Women 0-20 mm per hour. Raised ESR means anaemia, acute myocardial infarction, pulmonary tuberculosis, acute gout, burns and acute infections. It rises rapidly in rheumatic arthritis and chronic renal diseases. ESR not raised means influenza, chronic focal dental infection, ectopic pregnancy, psychogenic disease. Decreased value of ESR means congestive cardiac failure and polycythemia vera. Knowing the ESR value is a very good means of prognosis and treatment of diseases.

Serum Cholesterol 150-250 mg percent; increased level means cardiovascular disease and atherosclerosis, obstructive jaundice, nephrosis, uncontrolled diabetes. Decreased levels means malabsorption, liver disorders, anemia, stress.

High Density Lipoprotein (HDL) Men-45 mg/100 ml Women-55 mg/100ml; increased values are for chronic liver disorders, decreased levels are associated with increased risk of coronary heart disease.

VLDL AND LDL VLDL cholesterol 25 to 50 percent VLDL is a major carrier of triglycerides (60-70 percent triglyceride, 10-15 percent cholesterol). Degradation of VLDL leads to major source of LDL.

Triglycerides 40-150 mg per cent Triglycerides actually produce energy for the body and excess of triglycerides get stored in adipose tissue. Increased levels show liver disease, hypothyroidism, not controlled diabetes and myocardial infarction. Decreased level means mal absorption.

Glucose tolerance test 70-100 mg per 100 ml; fasting Oral glucose tolerance test 110 mg percent; fasting 140 mg – two hours after Elevated blood sugar means acute myocardial infarction, diabetes, pituitary adenoma, pancreatitis and chronic liver disease. Lower glucose level means overdose of insulin, malnutrition, bacterial septicaemia and carcinoma of pancreas.

Serum Bilirubin 0.8 mg% range 0.2 to 0.8 mg% Increased levels mean heptacellular jaundice, viral hepatitis, cirrhosis of liver and some other reasons.

Blood Urea Nitrogen (BUN) 25-40 mg percent; increased level means impaired renal function, shock, diabetes, acute myocardial infarction, chronic gout and excessive protein intake. Decreased level shows liver failure, malnutrition and over hydration.

Uric acid 4-7 mg percent; increased level shows leukemia, metastatic cancer, starvation, chemotherapy for cancer, excessive radiation, diabetic ketosis.

Note: There are many other tests but are not relevant for layman purpose. Another thing to be noted by the patients is that they find the colour of their urine or stool changed after they take medicines. One should not get alarmed due to this. Drugs containing iron, bismuth, lead, aspirin, aluminum charcoal etc. lead to discolouration of stools. Vitamin B complex, C, drugs containing mercury, alcohol, furazolidone, nitrofurantoin, chloroquine, arsenicals etc. change the colour of urine.

LASTING OF DISEASES
(INVUBSTION/COMMUNICABILITY)

For a layman, it is essential to know how long a disease will continue after he or she takes drugs. Here is a short list of diseases with their duration. Disease incubation period or communicability:

Influenza 1 to 3 days

Dysentery (bacillary) 1 to 7 days till bacilli in stool

Typhoid 5 days till negative stool/urine report

Cholera 3 days

Smallpox 7 to 17 days

Mumps 2 to 3 weeks until the swelling subsides

Polio 7 to 14 days

Scabies 1 to 2 days till it is cured

Measles 1 to 3 days one week

Albert Einstein has said, 'The significant problems we face cannot be solved at the same level of thinking we were at when we created them'.

This is very true that times change and with the time, the views and our thinking also changes. But in the case of up keeping the health, we have not changed much. The rules of our routine can never change. The bathing, washing, use of cosmetics, the need for oxygen, exercise, good food, observing rules about age-wise life and other health factors can never change. The changes are in accordance with the traditional and environmental conditions in the particular regions one lives in. All over the world, people follow traditional rules of health as seen in the families and as read in the ancient therapy literature of the land. These rules were framed thousands of years ago and naturally are of utmost value in the milieu prevailing at the time of writing books. These ideas were found very useful for health and beauty. As the time passed, beauty-scholars wrote many other books but the basic idea and methods of keeping a good beautiful body is almost the same. We have changed some of the methods but the idea of 'be beautiful and look beautiful' has been the same.

The spiritual dimension makes us aware that we have a relation of body with our soul or internal force. So far as we accept the idea of spiritual being, our health and beauty will not get worsened. From time to time, we need to meditate, offer prayers, and make offerings to God. Deep concentration in good literature of health and in good music will satisfy the hunger of our soul.

Bibliography

1. The Organon—S. Hanemann; Diseases of skin—Fredrick M. Dearborn
2. Introduction to Dermatology—Norman Walker and G.H. Percival
3. Textbook of Dermatology—Ramji Gupta and R. K. Manchanda
4. Select your Remedy—R.B.Bishamber Das
5. Domestic Physician—Constantine Herring
6. Bhojan Dwara Chikitsa—Ganesh Narayan Chauhan
7. Ayurvedic Remedies—T.L. Devraj
8. Arogya Parkash—Vaidhraj Ram Narayan Sharma
9. Ayurveda, the Science of Healing—Vasant Lad
10. Yogasans—Sant Vaid ji
11. Principles and Art of Cure by Homoeopathy—H. L. Roberts
12. Hair, Skin and Beauty Care—Blossom Kochhar
13. From Old Age to Youth—Satyavarta Sidhantalnkar
14. Mega-nutrients for your Nerves H.L. Newbold; Oral Diseases—Shiv Dua
15. Neck pain, Cervical Spondylosis—Shiv Dua
16. Homoeopathic Self Healing Guide—Shiv Dua
17. Hair Care—Shiv Dua